POCKET GUIDE

S0-BCZ-547

FOR USE WITH
MEDICAL ASSISTING

Administrative and Clinical Procedures with Anatomy and Physiology 6e

Kathryn A. Booth, RN-BSN, RMA (AMT), RPT, CPhT, MS
Total Care Programming, Inc.
Palm Coast, Florida

Leesa G. Whicker, BA, CMA (AAMA)
Central Piedmont Community College
Charlotte, North Carolina

Terri D. Wyman, CPC, CMRS
Baystate Wing Hospital
Palmer, Massachusetts

POCKET GUIDE FOR USE WITH MEDICAL ASSISTING, SIXTH EDITION

1 2 3 4 5 6 7 8 9 0 SCI/SCI 1 0 9 8 7 6

ISBN 978-1-259-73187-7
MHID 1-259-73187-1

Senior Vice President, Products & Markets: *Kurt L. Strand*
Vice President, General Manager, Products & Markets: *Marty Lange*
Vice President, Content Design & Delivery: *Kimberly Meriwether David*
Managing Director: *Chad Grall*
Executive Brand Manager: *William Lawrensen*
Director, Product Development: *Rose Koos*
Senior Product Developer: *Christine Scheid*
Product Developer: *Michelle Gaseor*
Marketing Manager: *Harper Christopher*
Digital Product Analyst: *Katherine Ward*
Director, Content Design & Delivery: *Linda Avenarius*
Program Manager: *Angela R. FitzPatrick*
Content Project Managers: *April R. Southwood/Brent dela Cruz*
Buyer: *Jennifer Pickel*
Design: *Srdjan Savanovic*
Content Licensing Specialists: *Lori Hancock/Lorraine Buczek*
Cover Image: Lung: © Nucleus Medical Media; Taking the temperature: © M. Constantini/PhotoAlto; Schedule Practice Fusion: © Practice Fusion; Urine testing canister with rainbow squares: © McGraw-Hill Education; Desk: © MuzzyLane; Gloved hands: © McGraw-Hill Education/Mark A. Dierker, photographer
Compositor: *SPi Global*
Printer: *Strategic Content Imaging*

All credits appearing on page or at the end of the book are considered to be an extension of the copyright page.

mheducation.com/highered

Contents

Section 1: Administrative

Section 2: Clinical

Section 3: Laboratory

Section 4: General

Appendixes

Part 2

Page 83, 2015 Recommended Immunizations for Children from 7 Through 18 Years Old: Reprinted courtesy of the Centers for Disease Control and Prevention.

Page 84, 2015 Recommended Immunizations for Adults: By Age: Reprinted courtesy of the Centers for Disease Control and Prevention.

Page 85, 2015 Recommended Immunizations for Children from Birth Through 6 Years Old: Reprinted courtesy of the Centers for Disease Control and Prevention.

Pages 139–140, Calories Burned During Activities: Source: Dietary Guidelines for Americans 2005, US Department of Health and Human Services, US Department of Agriculture, www.healthierus.gov/dietaryguidelines.

Page 140, Food Label Terms: Reprinted courtesy of the US Department of Agriculture and US Department of Health and Human Services.

Page 141, Saturated Fat and Cholesterol Sources: Reprinted courtesy of the US Department of Agriculture.

Page 142, Serving Sizes: Reprinted courtesy of the US Department of Agriculture and US Department of Health and Human Services.

Pages 145–147, USDA 2010 Dietary Guidelines Key Recommendations: Adapted from "Dietary Guidelines for Americans 2010," US Department of Agriculture and US Department of Health and Human Services, www.dietaryguidelines.gov.

Page 148, Vitamins: Reprinted courtesy of the US Department of Agriculture.

1 Administrative

Schedule Management

Scheduling Systems

- **Advance scheduling**—patients are given appointments well in advance
- **Cluster scheduling**—similar types of appointments are clustered together during the day or week
- **Combination scheduling**—a combination of more than one scheduling system is used
- **Double booking**—two or more patients are scheduled for the same appointment slot
- **Modified-wave**—similar to wave scheduling; patients arrive at scheduled intervals during an hour, allowing time to catch up before the next hour begins
- **Open-hours**—patients arrive at their own convenience and are seen on a first-come, first-served basis
- **Time-specified**—each patient is given an individual appointment time
- **Wave**—several patients are given the same appointment time beginning on the hour and are seen in the order they arrive; determine the number of patients per hour by dividing the hour by the average appointment length

Patient Information Needed to Schedule an Appointment

- Patient's full name
- Contact telephone numbers
- Purpose of the visit

Scheduling Emergency Appointments

- Determine if an acute condition is an emergency based on office guidelines.
- If unsure, ask the provider for instructions.
- Adjust the schedule as necessary to accommodate patients with emergencies.
- You may need to reschedule some patient appointments.
- Let waiting patients know there is an emergency without giving details.

Scheduling Surgery

Inpatient surgery

1. Check the physician's schedule to see when she is scheduled to be in the operating room.
2. Call the operating room secretary. Give the procedure required, the name of the surgeon, the time involved, and the preferred date and hour.
3. Provide the patient's name (including birth name, if appropriate), address, telephone number, age, gender, patient identification number, and insurance information.
4. Call the admissions office. Arrange for the patient to be admitted on the day of surgery or the day before as indicated.
5. Have the patient complete any preadmission forms the hospital requires.
6. Confirm the surgery and the patient's arrival time 1 business day before surgery.

Outpatient surgery

Scheduling outpatient surgery is similar to inpatient surgery but is often booked at a surgi-center or hospital outpatient surgery area.

Typical Lengths of Common Office Procedures

Complete PE	30–60 minutes
New patient visit	30–45 minutes
Follow-up office visit	5–15 minutes
Emergency office visit	15–20 minutes
Prenatal exam	15 minutes
Pap smear and pelvic exam	15–30 minutes
Minor in-office surgery	30 minutes
Suture removal	10–20 minutes

Written and Electronic Communication

Basic Rules of Writing

Capitalization

Use capital letters for the following:

- All proper names
- All titles, positions, or indications of family relation when preceding a proper name or in place of a proper noun
- Days of the week, months, and holidays
- Names of organizations and membership designations
- Racial, religious, and political designations
- Adjectives, nouns, and verbs that are derived from proper nouns
- Specific addresses and geographic locations
- Sums of money written in legal or business documents
- Titles, headings of books, magazines, and newspapers

Numbers

Use numerals

- In general writing, when the number is 11 or greater.
- With abbreviations and symbols.

- When discussing laboratory results or statistics.
- When referring to specific sums of money.
- When using a series of numbers in a sentence.

Tips

- Use commas when numerals have more than three digits.
- Do not use commas when referring to account numbers, page numbers, or policy numbers.
- Use a hyphen with numerals to indicate a range.

Plurals

- Add *s* or *es* to most singular nouns.
- With medical terms ending in *is*, drop the *is* and add *es*.
- With terms ending in *um,* drop the *um* and add *a*.
- With terms ending in *us,* drop the *us* and add *i*.
- With terms ending in *a,* keep the *a* and add *e*.

Possessives

To show ownership or relation to another noun, follow the rules below.

- For singular nouns, add an apostrophe and an *s*.
- For plural nouns that do not end in an *s*, add an apostrophe and an *s*.
- For plural nouns that end in an *s*, just add an apostrophe.

Word division

Divide

- According to pronunciation.
- In compound words, between the two words from which they derive.

- In hyphenated compound words, at the hyphen.
- After a prefix.
- Before a suffix.
- Between two consonants that appear between vowels.
- Before *-ing* unless the last consonant is doubled; in that case, divide before the second consonant.

Do not divide

- Suffixes such as *-sion, -tial,* and *-gion.*
- A word so that only one letter is left on a line.

Letter Styles

- **Full-block**—all lines are flush left. May use mixed or open punctuation
- **Modified-block**—similar to full-block except that the dateline, complimentary closing, and signature block are aligned at or slightly to the right of the center of the page; may use mixed or open punctuation
- **Modified-block with indented paragraphs**—identical to modified-block except that paragraphs are indented 1/2 inch; may use mixed or open punctuation
- **Simplified**—modification of full-block with omitted salutation and complimentary closing; includes a subject line and uses open punctuation

Parts of a Letter

- **Margin**—the space around the edges of a form or letter that are left blank; the business standard is 1 inch
- **Letterhead**—the preprinted portion of business stationery
- **Dateline**—the month, day, year (for example, July 5, 20xx); place it approximately three lines below the letterhead on preprinted stationery

- **Inside address**—the name and address of the person to whom the letter is being sent; place it two to four lines down from the date; include the following:
  - Courtesy title (Dr., Mr., Mrs., Ms.)
  - Company name if applicable
  - Numerals for street address, except the single numbers one through nine
    - Spell out numerical names of streets if less than 10.
    - Spell out the words *Street, Drive,* etc.
  - Full city name
  - Two-letter USPS state abbreviation
    - Leave one space between the state and zip code.
- **Salutation**—written greeting such as *Dear*
- **Subject line**—information that brings the subject of the letter to the reader's attention
  - Place on second line below the salutation.
  - Place flush with left margin, indented five spaces, or centered depending on letter style used.
  - Include two or three words.
  - Set in all capital letters.
- **Body**—single-spaced text that is the largest part of the letter
  - Begin it two lines below the salutation or subject line.
  - Double-space between paragraphs.
- **Complimentary closing**—written closing; *Sincerely, Very truly yours,* and *Best regards* are acceptable business closings
  - Include it two lines below last line of the body.
  - Capitalize the first letter only.
- **Signature block**—signature that includes the writer's name and business title
  - Align it with the complimentary closing.

- Include it three to four lines below the closing.
- Place the writer's name on the first line.
- Place the writer's business title on the second line.
- **Identification line**—the writer's initials (in CAPS) followed by a colon or slash and the typist's initials (lowercase)
  - Include it flush left.
  - Place it two lines below the signature block.
- **Notations**—the number of enclosures included with the letter and the names of people receiving copies of the letter
  - Place it one or two lines below the identification line.

Writing Tips

- Know the type of person to whom you are writing.
- Know the purpose of the letter.
- Be concise, clear, brief, and specific.
- Do not use unnecessary words.
- Use the active voice except when softening the tone of the letter.
- Check spelling, grammar, and accuracy of dates and numbers.

Tips on Electronic Communication

- Regardless of the format, remember you are writing as a representative of the practice.
- Before sending electronic communication to a patient, be sure the appropriate consent is on file.
- If a template is used, make sure all required changes are made so that the communication contains information intended solely for the person receiving the e-mail.
- Follow office policy regarding "dos and don'ts" for e-mail communications.
- Check your office e-mail inbox frequently, deleting unwanted messages.

- Never open unidentifiable e-mails.
- Set up a subfolder for communications that must be kept indefinitely.
- Save all e-mail responses containing PHI.

Charting and Documenting

6 Cs of Charting

- **Client's words**—record the exact words.
- **Clarity**—use precise language.
- **Completeness**—fill out the entire form.
- **Conciseness**—be brief and to the point.
- **Chronological order**—date entries in order.
- **Confidentiality**—protect the patient's privacy.

Ensuring That the Provider Can Find the Most Recent Patient Information

- Record all findings from exams and tests as soon as they are available.
- Document telephone calls by recording the date and time of the call, who initiated it, the information discussed, and any conclusions or results.
- Establish a procedure for retrieving a paper file quickly in case of emergency.

Coding Guidelines or Steps

Code Linkage

The procedural code should be linked to a diagnosis code. A code review should ensure that

- Codes are appropriate for the patient profile.

- Each code is billable.
- A clear and correct link exists between each procedure and at least one listed diagnosis.
- Payer's rules about diagnosis and procedures are followed.
- Documentation in the patient's medical record supports the reported services.
- Reported services comply with all insurance and governmental regulations.

Global Period

The global period is the period of time that is covered for follow-up care. The length of time will vary depending on the type of procedure performed.

Diagnostic Coding

Alphabetic index

- An index of the disease and condition descriptions in the Tabular List
- An index in table format of drugs and chemicals that cause poisoning
- An index of external causes of injury, such as accidents

Tabular list

- Alphanumeric listing of code descriptions from Alpha Index
- Explicit coding instructions are found here.

Code structure

- ICD-9 codes are made up of three, four, or five characters and a description.
- ICD-10 codes (10/1/2015) are made up of three to seven characters and a description.

- The basic structure, known as the rubric, is three characters for both ICD-9 and ICD-10.
- Adding a fourth and/or fifth character makes the ICD-9 code more specific.
- Optional fourth through seventh characters are mandatory if available for an ICD-10 code to increase its specificity.

Coding conventions

These symbols provide guidelines for using the code set.

- **NOS**—not otherwise specified
- **NEC**—not elsewhere classified
- [ ] Brackets—used around synonyms, alternative wordings, or explanations
- **( )** Parentheses—used around descriptions that do not affect the code selection
- : Colon—used in the Tabular List after an incomplete term that needs one of the terms that follow to make it assignable to a given category
- } Brace—encloses a series of terms, each of which is modified by the statement that appears to the right of the brace
- ***Includes***—indicates that the entries following it refine the content of a preceding entry
- ***Excludes 1***—indicates that an entry is not classified as part of the preceding code and the two codes are never coded together
- ***Excludes 2***—indicates that the entry is not part of the preceding code; however, if both diagnoses exist, they may both be coded
- ***Use additional code***—indicates that an additional code should be used, if information is provided
- ***Code first underlying disease***—appears when the category is not to be used as the primary diagnosis

Translating Patient and Provider Words into Codes for Insurance Claims

The Patient Says	The Physician Documents	CPT Code	HCPCS Code	ICD-10 Code
1. I have a constant cough but can't move the mucus. My chest feels "full."	T 99.2 P 80 and reg BP 130/82 EENT: PEERLA Chest reveals wheezing & "wet" breath sounds Order CBC /w diff and chest X-ray Rx: Z-Pak for 1 week To call in progress report in 3 days Dx: Acute Bronchitis	(Exam) 99213 (C-XR) 71020 (CBC) 85025	None	(Bronchitis) J20.9
2. I fell off a ladder getting off the roof at home. My left ankle is swollen and killing me.	34 y/o white male in moderate distress. EENT: PEERLA Chest clear. Abdomen nontender LLE swollen and angulated below knee Other extremities normal LLE X-ray reveals bimalleolar (nondisplaced) fracture Closed Fx with cast app and crutches No weight-bearing. F/U with Ortho Percocet #10 prn pain	(ED Exam) 99283 (X-ray) 73610 (Fx reduction) 27808	(Crutches) E0112	(Fx) S82.845 (Fall) W11xxxA (Location) Y92.00
3. My heart races and I have trouble catching my breath. I get really light-headed when it occurs.	42 y/o female in mild distress. Obviously dyspneic and tachycardic T 98.2 P 225 BP 150/90 ECG shows A-fib and PATs Admit for OBS. Holter monitor, CX-R, chem panel to be performed	(Admit) 99222 (ECG) 93000 (CX-R) 71020 (Holter) 93224 (Labs) 88050	None	(PAT) I47.1 (A-fib) I48.0 (Hypothyroid) E03.9

11

Locating an ICD (diagnostic) code

CRITICAL PROCEDURE STEPS

1. Locate the patient's diagnosis.
2. Find the diagnosis in the Alphabetic Index.
3. Locate the code from the Alphabetic Index in the Tabular List.
4. Pick the most specific code available.
5. Record the code on the insurance claim form.

External cause codes

- Identify the external causes of injury or poisoning and/or the location where the accident took place.
- Always supplement a code that identifies the injury or condition.
- Used in collecting public health information

Health status codes

Z Codes

- Identify encounters for reasons other than illness or injury
- May be used as a primary code or as an additional code

Tabular List Organization for ICD-10

Chapter	Categories
1. Certain Infectious and Parasitic Diseases	A00–B99.9
2. Neoplasms	C00–D49.9

Chapter	Categories
3. Diseases of the Blood and Blood-Forming Organs	D50–D89.9
4. Endocrine, Nutritional and Metabolic Diseases	E00–E89.89
5. Mental and Behavioral Disorders	F01–F99
6. Diseases of the Nervous System	G00–G99.8
7. Diseases of the Eye and Adnexa	H00–H59.89
8. Diseases of the Ear and Mastoid Process	H60–H95.89
9. Diseases of the Circulatory System	I00–I99.9
10. Diseases of the Respiratory System	J00–J99
11. Diseases of the Digestive System	K00–K94.39
12. Diseases of the Skin and Subcutaneous Tissue	L00–L99
13. Diseases of the Musculoskeletal System and Connective Tissue	M00–M99.9
14. Diseases of the Genitourinary System	N00–N99.89
15. Pregnancy, Childbirth, and the Puerperium	O00–O9A.53
16. Certain Conditions Originating in the Perinatal Period	P00–P96.9
17. Congenital Malformations, Deformations, and Chromosomal Abnormalities	Q00–Q99.9

continued

Chapter	Categories
18. Symptoms, Signs, and Abnormal Clinical and Laboratory Findings	R00–R99
19. Injury, Poisoning, and Certain Other Consequences of External Causes	S00–T98
20. External Causes of Morbidity	V00–Y99.9
21. Factors Influencing Health Status and Contact with Health Services	Z00–Z99.89

Procedural Coding

Add-on codes

These codes are used for procedures that are carried out in addition to another procedure. They are noted by a + sign in front of the CPT code.

Code modifiers

Modifiers show that some special circumstance applies to the service or procedure the practitioner performed.

Code ranges

Evaluation and Management	99201–99499
Anesthesiology	00100–01999, 99100–99140
Surgery	10021–69990
Radiology	70010–79999
Pathology and Laboratory	80047–89398
Medicine	90281–99199, 99500–99607

E and M codes

These codes help determine how to code differing levels of medical and provider services. Guidelines determining level of service include the following:

- The extent of the patient history taken
- The extent of the exam conducted
- The complexity of the medical decision making
- Whether the patient is new or established
- The location of service

Locating a CPT code

CRITICAL PROCEDURE STEPS

1. Check the patient's record for services performed.
2. Look up the procedure in the CPT Alphabetic Index.
3. Verify the chosen code in the Tabular List.
4. Determine appropriate modifiers.
5. Record the code on the insurance claim form.

Computer and Equipment Troubleshooting

Before calling a service agent:

- Check the simplest causes (power supply, equipment turned on, cables connected properly, etc.).
- Test the machine to see what it is failing to do.
- Write down any error messages.
- Check the equipment manual for a troubleshooting guide.

Cultural Concerns

Effective Communication

1. When it is necessary to use a translator, direct the conversation or instruction to the patient.
2. Direct demonstrations to the patient of what to do, such as putting on an exam gown.
3. Confirm with the translator that the patient has understood the instruction or demonstration.
4. Allow the translator to be present during the exam if that is the patient's preference.
5. If the patient understands some English, speak slowly, use simple language, and demonstrate instructions whenever possible.

Meeting the Need for Privacy

1. Before the procedure, thoroughly explain to the patient or translator the reason for disrobing. Indicate that you will allow the patient privacy and ample time to undress.
2. If the patient is reluctant, reassure him that the provider respects the need for privacy and will look at only what is necessary for the exam.
3. Provide extra drapes if you think doing so will make the patient feel more comfortable.
4. If the patient is still reluctant, discuss the problem with the provider, who may be able to negotiate a compromise with the patient.
5. During the procedure, ensure that the patient is undraped only as much as necessary.
6. Whenever possible, minimize the amount of time the patient remains undraped.

Cultural Differences

Filing Medical Records

Filing Steps

- **Inspecting (conditioning)**—prepare for filing
- **Indexing**—assign name or number to the file
- **Coding**—mark the file to identify it
- **Sorting**—alphabetically or numerically
- **Storing**—properly place the document or file

Filing Guidelines

- Be familiar with file contents.
- Keep the file neat.
- Do not crowd the folder or file drawer.
- Position file guides 5 inches apart.
- Cross-reference when appropriate.
- File regularly.
- Store files in their proper location.
- Train personnel to file appropriately.
- Periodically evaluate the filing system.

Locating Misplaced Paper Files

When searching for a misplaced paper file:

- Determine where the file was last seen.
- Retrace your steps.
- Check neighboring files in the cabinet.
- Check underneath the cabinet for lost files.
- Recheck the pile to be filed.
- Check similar indexes.
- Check the provider's office.
- Check with coworkers.
- Check first name filing.
- Look for files that stand out from others.
- Determine if someone else could have picked up the file.
- Have someone check behind you.
- Straighten the office and check for the lost file.

Rules for Alphabetic Filing

Rules

1. Treat each part of a patient's name as a separate unit, and look at the units in this order: last name, first name, middle initial, and any subsequent names or initials.
2. Treat a prefix, such as the *O'* in *O'Hara,* as part of the name, not as a separate unit. Ignore variations in spacing, punctuation, and capitalization. Treat prefixes such as *De La, Mac, Saint,* and *St.* exactly as they are spelled.
3. Treat hyphenated names as a single unit. Disregard the hyphen.
4. A title, such as *Dr.* or *Major,* or a seniority term, such as *Jr.* or *3d,* should be treated as the last filing unit to distinguish names that are otherwise identical.

Examples

- Stephen Jacobson

Unit 1	Unit 2	Unit 3	Unit 4
Jacobson	Stephen		

- Stephen Brent Jacobson

Unit 1	Unit 2	Unit 3	Unit 4
Jacobson	Stephen	Brent	

- Victor P. De La Cruz

Unit 1	Unit 2	Unit 3	Unit 4
Delacruz	Victor	P	

- Jean-Marie Vigneau

Unit 1	Unit 2	Unit 3	Unit 4
Vigneau	Jeanmarie		

- Dr. George B. Diaz

Unit 1	Unit 2	Unit 3	Unit 4
Diaz	George	B	Dr

- Major George B. Diaz

Unit 1	Unit 2	Unit 3	Unit 4
Diaz	George	B	Major

- James R. Foster, Jr.

Unit 1	Unit 2	Unit 3	Unit 4
Foster	James	R	Jr

Rules for Numeric Filing

1. Medical record numbers are generally split into three sections: for example, 111-222-333.
2. In consecutive digit filing, each section is filed as a whole number, moving left to right.
3. In middle digit filing, each section is filed as a whole number, starting in the middle section, then the left, and finally the right section.
4. In terminal digit filing, each section is filed as a whole number starting at the right and moving to the left.

The table that follows illustrates how the example MRN 111-222-333 would be filed using each of the three numeric filing types.

Filing System	Unit 1	Unit 2	Unit 3
Consecutive digit	111	222	333
Middle digit	222	111	333
Terminal digit	333	222	111

Insurance Tips

Claims Process Overview

The general steps in the claims process are

- Gathering and recording patient information.
- Verifying the patient's insurance information.
- Recording procedures and services.
- Determining a diagnosis for each procedure or service.
- Filing claims; recording insurance payments and adjustments.
- Billing patients and recording patient payments.

Completing a CMS-1500 Claim Form

CRITICAL PROCEDURE STEPS

The numbers below correspond to the numbered fields on the CMS-1500 form. When completing the form, you should enter the following:

1. Insurance type
1a. Insured's insurance ID number
2. Patient's name (last, first, middle initial)
3. Patient's birth date and sex
4. Insured's name or "Same" if patient and insured are the same
5. Patient's mailing address
6. Patient's relationship to the insured
7. Insured's mailing address
8. Leave blank; reserved for NUCC use
9. Name of any other insured party
9a. Policy number of other insured party
9b. Leave blank; reserved for NUCC use
9c. Leave blank; reserved for NUCC use
9d. Other insured's insurance plan
10. Information about the related cause of the condition
11. Insured's policy group number; enter "NONE" for Medicare
11a. Insured's date of birth and sex
11b. Other claim ID designated by NUCC, if applicable
11c. Insurance plan or program name
11d. Information about another insurance plan, if any
12. Patient or authorized representative signature and date

continued

13. Insured's signature
14. Date of current illness, injury, or pregnancy
15. Other date related to patient's condition or pregnancy if known; leave blank for Medicare
16. Dates patient unable to work
17. Name of the referring provider, or referring source; enter appropriate qualifier in space to left of provider name
17a. If required by payer, qualifier and other provider ID
17b. NPI
18. Dates the patient was hospitalized, if applicable
19. If required by payer, insert required additional claim information
20. Select whether any laboratory tests were done at an outside lab and insert charges, if any
21. ICD code or codes
22. Resubmission code and original reference number (if required by payer)
23. Prior authorization number if required
24A. Dates of service
24B. Place of service code
24C. Emergency (Y/N) (Medicaid only)
24D. CPT/HCPCS codes
24E. Diagnosis code reference (A–L) that applies to that procedure (up to 4 per procedure)
24F. Fee charged
24G. Number of days or units on which the service is provided
24H. Early and Periodic Screening, Diagnosis, and Treatment (Medicaid only)

24I. Secondary provider ID qualifier (in red block if required)

24J. Provider secondary ID (in red block if required); provider NPI in white block

25. Federal tax ID number (select whether SSN or EIN)

26. Patient account number assigned by provider office (if used)

27. Assignment of benefits (Y or N)

28. Total charge

29. Amount already paid

30. Leave blank; reserved for NUCC use

31. Provider signature and date

32. Name and address of service provider (if different from billing provider)

32a. Service provider NPI

33. Billing provider's name, address, telephone number

33a. Billing provider NPI

Determining Primary Coverage

- If the patient has only one policy, it is primary.
- If the patient has two plans, the one that has been in effect the longest is primary unless one plan is Medicare and the other is a supplement. In this case, Medicare is primary.
- If the patient is also covered as a dependent on another plan, the patient's plan is primary.

- If an employed patient has coverage under the employer's plan and additional coverage under a government-sponsored plan (such as Medicare or Medicaid), the employer's plan is primary.
- If a retired patient is covered by the plan of the spouse's employer and the spouse is still employed, the spouse's plan is primary.
- If a patient is a dependent child covered by both parents' plans and the parents are not separated or divorced, the primary plan is determined by which parent has the first birth date in the calendar year.
- If two or more plans cover the dependent children of separated or divorced parents who do not have joint custody of their children, the children's primary plan is determined in this order:
  - The plan of the custodial parent
  - The plan of the spouse of the custodial parent (if the parent has remarried)
  - The plan of the parent without custody

Elements of an EOB/EOP (Explanation of Benefits/ Payment)

- Name and identification number of the insured
- Name of the beneficiary
- Claim number
- Date, place, and type of service
- Amount billed by the practice
- Amount allowed
- Amount of subscriber liability

- Amount paid and included in the current payment
- A notation of any services not covered and an explanation of why they were not covered

Generating Clean Claims

Insurance claims may be rejected because of missing or invalid information:

- Service facility name and complete address
- Medicare or benefits assignments indicator
- Referring provider name or indicator
- Subscriber's birth date
- Information about secondary insurance
- Payer name and/or payer identifier
- Misspelling of patient or subscriber name

Inventory

Inventory Procedures Overview

1. Define your role and responsibility in managing supplies.
2. Create a formal supply list of all administrative and clinical supplies.
3. Start a file containing a list of vendors and their current catalogs.
4. Create a want list of products.
5. Make a file for supply invoices and completed order forms.
6. Devise an inventory system for each item.
7. Devise a system for flagging items that need to be ordered or have already been ordered.
8. Establish a regular inventory schedule.

9. Order on a regular schedule unless an item is needed immediately.
10. Complete the vendor's order form.
11. Place the order online or by telephone, fax, or e-mail.
12. When the order arrives, check the shipment against the original order form and record the amount received on the individual inventory card or page.
13. Check the invoice and sign and date it when the order is received.
14. Write a check to the vendor according to office policy.
15. Mail the check to the vendor and file the invoice with the original order and the packing slip.

Recording Supply Inventory

You should devise an inventory system for each item used in a medical office. Keep a card or sheet for each item with the following information:

- Date and quantity of each order
- Name and contact information of the vendor and sales representative
- Date each shipment was received
- Total cost and unit cost for the item
- Payment method used
- Results of periodic counts of the item
- Quantity expected to cover the office for a given period of time
- Reorder quantity

Medical Records

Contents

- Patient registration form (The basis for the patient financial record)
- Patient medical history
- Physical exam results
- Results of laboratory and other tests
- Records from other physicians and hospitals
- Doctor's diagnosis and treatment plan
- Operative reports, follow-up visits, telephone calls
- Consent forms
- Hospital discharge summary forms
- Patient correspondence
- Faxed information

Making Corrections in a Paper Medical Record

YOU SHOULD KNOW

- Correct errors without deception.
- Do not delete or cover the information.
- Draw a single line through the information.
- Write correct information above or below the line.
- Note why the correction was made if appropriate.
- Enter the date, the time, and your initials.

Preparing the (Paper) Record

CRITICAL PROCEDURE STEPS

1. Create a chart label according to practice policy. The label may contain the patient's first and last name or a medical record number.
2. Appropriately place the label on the folder.
3. Appropriately place the date label on the folder, updating the date if necessary.
4. If alpha or numeric labels are used, place a patient name label according to office policy.
5. Punch holes in the appropriate forms for placement in the patient's chart.
6. Place all forms in the appropriate sections of the patient's chart.

Types of Medical Records

Problem-oriented medical record

- **Database**—patient's history, initial interview information, findings and results of physical exam
- **Problem list**—each patient problem listed separately by number
- **Diagnostic and treatment plan**—laboratory and diagnostic tests and the physician's treatment plan
- **Progress notes**—notes on every condition or problem listed in the problem list

SOAP documentation

- *Subjective* data—the patient's description of his or her signs and symptoms
- *Objective* data—the provider's exam and test results

- *Assessment*—diagnosis or impression of a patient's diagnosis
- *Plan*—treatment options, chosen treatment, medications, tests, consultations, patient education, and follow-up

CHEDDAR documentation

- **C**: Chief complaint, presenting problems, subjective statements
- **H**: History; past medical, family, and social histories as well as the history of presenting problem (HPI) and any other contributing information
- **E**: Examination, including extent of body systems examined
- **D**: Details of problem and complaints
- **D**: Drugs and dosage; a list of current medications, including dosage and frequency
- **A**: Assessment of the diagnostic process and the impression (diagnosis) made by the physician
- **R**: Return visit information or referral, if applicable

Releasing the Record

YOU SHOULD KNOW

- Obtain a signed and newly dated release from the patient authorizing the transfer of information.
- Make photocopies of the original material.
- Send only those portions of the record covered by the release and only records originating from your facility.
- Do not send originals.
- Call the recipient to confirm that all materials were received.

Patient Care Partnership

Patient History

Elements of a Patient History

- **Personal data**—name, patient number, birth date, etc.
- **Chief complaint**—the reason the patient is being seen
- **History of present illness**—information about the chief complaint, including date of onset, what treatments the patient has undergone, and medications taken
- **Past medical history**—any and all health problems present and past
- **Family history**—health of the patient's family
- **Social and occupational history**—marital status, sexual behaviors and orientation, occupations, hobbies, use of chemical substances
- **Review of systems**—the provider's systematic review of each body system

Obtaining a Medical History

CRITICAL PROCEDURE STEPS

1. Review the patient history form and plan your interview.
2. Take the patient to a private room, identify yourself, and correctly identify the patient.
3. Explain the medical history form.
4. Ask appropriate questions using open-ended sentences.
5. Accurately document the patient's responses.
6. Offer to answer any questions.
7. Sign or initial the patient history form and file in the patient's chart.
8. Inform the provider that you have completed the medical history form.

Patient Interviewing Skills

- **Effective listening**—use active listening skills; provide feedback
- **Nonverbal clues and body language**—be aware of tone of voice, facial expression, and body language
- **Broad knowledge base**—stay abreast of new techniques, diseases, and symptoms
- **Summarizing**—when recording information, repeat back a summary of information to the patient

Patient Responsibilities

Each patient has a responsibility to do the following:

- Provide information about past illnesses, hospitalizations, medications, and other matters related to her health status
- Participate in decision making by asking for additional information about her health status or treatment when she does not fully understand information and instructions
- Provide healthcare agencies with a copy of her written advance directive if she has one
- Inform physicians and other caregivers if she anticipates problems in following a prescribed treatment
- Follow the practitioner's orders for treatment
- Provide healthcare agencies with necessary information for insurance claims and work with the healthcare facility to make arrangements to pay fees when necessary

Payment Information Found in a Financial Record

Each patient financial record should include the information necessary to file the patient's insurance and bill the patient for any appropriate balance. When checking in a patient, make sure you review the chart for the following information:

- Address and phone number
- Insurance information
- Name of the person responsible for the payment

Patient-Centered Medical Home (PCHM)

Promising model to improve patient care and medical outcomes. Its attributes:

- Comprehensive care
- Patient-centered
- Coordinated care
- Accessible service
- Quality and safety

USPS State Abbreviations

Alabama AL

Alaska AK

Arizona AZ

Arkansas AR

California CA

Colorado CO

Connecticut CT

Delaware DE

District of Columbia DC

Florida FL

Georgia GA

Hawaii HI

Idaho ID

Illinois IL

Indiana IN

Iowa IA

Kansas KS

Kentucky KY

Louisiana LA

Maine ME

Maryland MD

Massachusetts MA

Michigan MI

Minnesota MN

Mississippi MS

Missouri MO

Montana MT

Nebraska NE

Nevada NV

New Hampshire NH

New Jersey NJ

New Mexico NM

New York NY

North Carolina NC

North Dakota ND

Ohio OH

Oklahoma OK

Oregon OR

Pennsylvania PA

Puerto Rico PR

Rhode Island RI

South Carolina SC

South Dakota SD

Tennessee TN

Texas TX

Utah UT

Vermont VT

Virginia VA

Washington WA

West Virginia WV

Wisconsin WI

Wyoming WY

2 Clinical

Ambulation

Crutch Gaits

Four point

1. Move the right crutch forward.
2. Move the left foot forward to the level of the left crutch.
3. Move the left crutch forward.
4. Move the right foot forward to the level of the right crutch.

Three point

1. Move both crutches and the affected leg forward.
2. Move the unaffected leg forward while weight is balanced on both crutches.

Two point

1. Move the left crutch and the right foot forward at the same time.
2. Move the right crutch and the left foot forward at the same time.

Swing-to

1. Move both crutches forward at the same time.
2. Lift the body and swing to the crutches.
3. End with the tripod position again.

Swing-through

1. Move both crutches forward.
2. Move the body and swing past the crutches.

Teaching a Patient to Use Crutches

PATIENT EDUCATION TIPS

1. Before educating the patient, verify the physician's order.
2. Explain the procedure to the patient.
3. Have the patient stand erect, looking straight ahead.
4. Have the patient place the crutch tips 2 to 6 inches in front of and 4 to 6 inches to the side of each foot.
5. Ensure a 2-inch gap between the axilla and the axillary bar.
6. Teach the patient to get up from a chair.
7. Teach the patient the required gait.
8. Teach the patient to ascend stairs.
9. Teach the patient to descend stairs.

Using crutches: general guidelines

YOU SHOULD KNOW

- Do not lean on crutches.
- Report any tingling or numbness in the arms, hands, or shoulders.
- Support body weight with the hands.
- Always stand erect to prevent muscle strain.
- Look straight ahead when walking.

- Move the crutches not more than 6 inches at a time to maintain good balance.
- Check the crutch tips regularly for wear and replace as needed.
- Check the crutch tips for wetness; dry the tips if they are wet.
- Check all wing nuts and bolts for tightness.
- Wear flat, well-fitting, nonskid shoes.
- Remove throw rugs and other unsecured articles from traffic areas.
- Report any unusual pain in the affected leg.

Teaching a Patient to Use a Walker

PATIENT EDUCATION TIPS
Walking

1. Instruct the patient to step into the walker.
2. Have the patient place her hands on the handgrips.
3. Make sure the patient's feet are far enough apart to provide a stable base.
4. Have the patient move the walker forward about 6 inches.
5. Instruct the patient to move one leg forward and then the other.
6. Instruct the patient to move the walker forward again to continue walking.

PATIENT EDUCATION TIPS

Sitting

1. Have the patient turn her back to the bed or chair.
2. Instruct the patient to take short, careful steps backward until she feels the bed or chair at the back of her legs.
3. Have the patient keep the walker in front of herself, let go of the walker, and place both hands on the bed or chair arms or seat.
4. Instruct the patient to balance herself on her arms while lowering herself slowly to the bed or chair.
5. If the patient has an injured or affected leg, she should keep it forward while bending her unaffected leg and lowering her body to the chair or bed.

Bandages

Circular

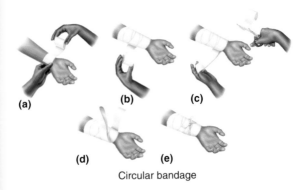

(a)

(b)

(c)

(d)

(e)

Circular bandage

Figure Eight

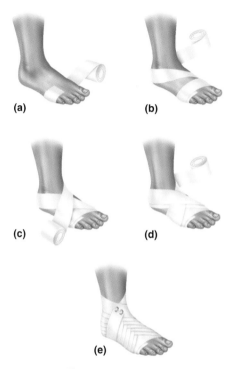

(a)

(b)

(c)

(d)

(e)

Figure eight bandage

Fingertip

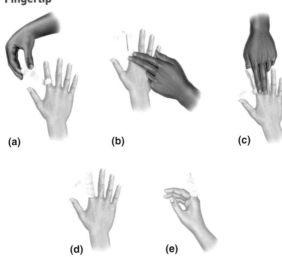

(a) **(b)** **(c)**

(d) **(e)**

Fingertip bandage

Sling

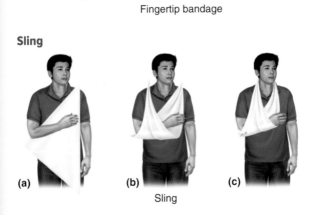

(a) **(b)** **(c)**

Sling

40

Triangular (Cravat)

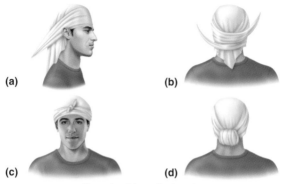

(a)

(b)

(c)

(d)

Cravat or triangular bandage

Biohazard Waste Disposal

Contaminated Paper Waste

CRITICAL PROCEDURE STEPS

1. Wear gloves.
2. Dispose of contaminated waste in an approved container.
3. Never dump the contents of one biohazardous waste container into another.
4. When the container is full, secure the inner liner and place the entire container in the appropriate area for biohazardous waste.
5. Remove gloves and wash your hands.

Sharps

CRITICAL PROCEDURE STEPS

1. Wear gloves.
2. Hold the object by the blunt end.
3. Drop the object directly into the approved container.

   If you are using an evacuation system, drop the entire evacuation system into an approved container.
4. Do not bend, break, or recap a needle.
5. Activate safety devices immediately after use.
6. Replace a container when it is two-thirds full.
7. Follow office procedure when disposing of containers.
8. Remove gloves and wash your hands.

Drug Abuse

Symptoms Associated with Abused Drugs

Drug Names/Type	Symptoms, Effects
Amphetamines/ stimulants	Altered mental status, from confusion to paranoia; hyperactivity, then exhaustion; insomnia; loss of appetite
Anabolic steroids	Irritability, aggression, nervousness, male-pattern baldness
Barbiturates/ sedatives	Slowed thinking, slowed reflexes, slowed respiration, loss of anxiety

Drug Names/Type	Symptoms, Effects
Benzodiazepines/sedatives	Poor coordination, drowsiness, increased self-confidence
Cocaine/stimulant	Alternating euphoria and apprehension, intense craving for more of the drug
Ecstasy/psychoactive	Confusion, depression, anxiety, paranoia, increased heart rate and blood pressure
GHB/depressants	Slow pulse and breathing, lowered blood pressure, drowsiness, poor concentration
Inhalants	Stimulation, intoxication, hearing loss, arm or leg spasms
LSD/hallucinogen	Heightened sense of awareness, grandiose hallucinations, mystical experiences, flashbacks
Marijuana, cannabinoids, hashish	Altered thought processes, distorted sense of time and self, impaired short-term memory
Opium, morphine, codeine/opiate narcotics	Decreased level of consciousness, detachment, drowsiness, impaired judgment
PCP/hallucinogen	Decreased awareness of surroundings, hallucinations, poor perception of time and distance, possible overdose and death

Ear Irrigation

CRITICAL PROCEDURE STEPS

1. Identify the patient and explain the procedure.
2. Check the physician's order.
3. Compare the solution with the order three times.
4. Wash your hands and put on gloves, a gown, and a face shield.
5. Look in the patient's ear to determine if cerumen or a foreign body is present.
6. Assemble the supplies.
7. Warm the solution to body temperature.
8. Have the patient sit or lie down, with the affected ear facing you.
9. Place a towel over the patient's shoulder and have her hold the basin under her ear.
10. Pour the solution into another basin.
11. If necessary, gently clean the patient's outer ear.
12. Fill the irrigating syringe with the solution.
13. Straighten the ear canal by pulling upward and outward for adults or down and back for infants and children.
14. Holding the tip of the syringe ½ inch from the ear canal, slowly instill the solution into the ear.
15. Refill the syringe and continue irrigation until the canal is cleaned or the solution is used up.
16. Dry the external ear with a cotton ball, and leave a clean cotton ball loosely in place for 5 to 10 minutes (if ordered).

17. If the patient becomes dizzy, allow her time to regain balance before standing.
18. Properly dispose of used disposable supplies.
19. Remove your gloves, gown, and face shield, and wash your hands.
20. Record in the patient's chart the procedure and result, the amount of solution used, the time of administration, and the ear(s) irrigated.
21. Put on gloves and clean the equipment and room according to OSHA guidelines.

ECGs

Artifacts

AC interference

- Cause: The electrocardiograph picks up small amounts of electric current given off by other pieces of equipment in the room.

- Example:

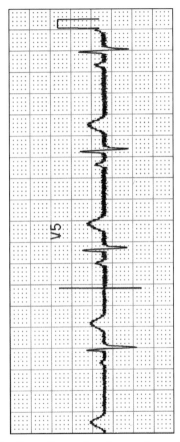

- Solution: Turn off or unplug other appliances in the room.

Flat line

- Cause: There may be a loose or disconnected wire or two of the wires may have been switched. A flat line may indicate cardiac arrest.

- Example: V6 lead

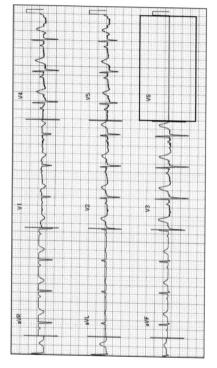

- Solution: Assess the patient's pulse and respirations first; then check all lead connections.

Somatic interference

- Cause: Muscle movement
- Example:

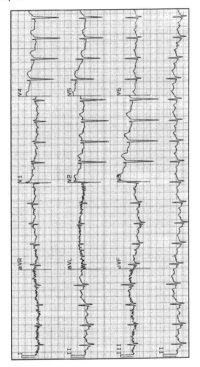

- Solution: Remind the patient to remain still and refrain from talking. If the patient is cold, offer him a blanket. If the patient is unable to stop a tremor, place the limb electrodes closer to the trunk of the body.

Wandering baseline

- Causes: Somatic interference, mechanical problems, and improper electrode application
- Example:

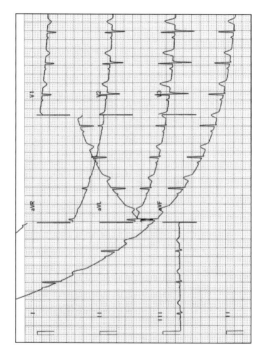

- Solution: Remind the patient to remain still, clean any oil or lotions from the skin before applying electrodes, check the electrodes and reapply if necessary, uncross any crossed wires, and reposition any dangling wires.

Critical Dysrhythmias

When performing an ECG, recognizing critical dysrhythmias is essential. The following pages illustrate atrial fibrillation, premature ventricular contractions, and ventricular fibrillation.

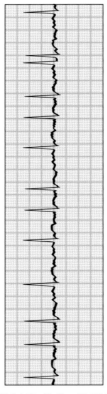

Atrial Fibrillation (A-Fib)

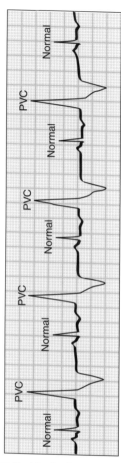

Premature Ventricular Contractions (PVCs)

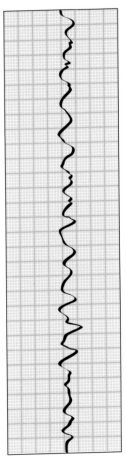

Ventricular Fibrillation (V-Fib)

Lead Placement

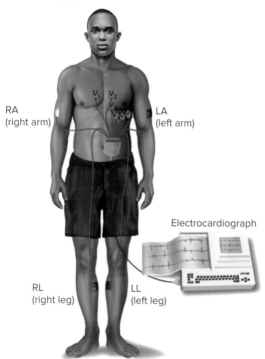

RA
(right arm)

LA
(left arm)

RL
(right leg)

LL
(left leg)

Electrocardiograph

Parts of the ECG

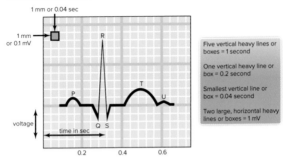

Five vertical heavy lines or boxes = 1 second

One vertical heavy line or box = 0.2 second

Smallest vertical line or box = 0.04 second

Two large, horizontal heavy lines or boxes = 1 mV

The ECG paper is standardized and includes heavy lines that allow measurement of both time and voltage. Note that each small box is either 0.1 mV in voltage or 0.04 second in time.

P wave

- Appearance—small, upward curve
- Represents—SA node impulse, wave of depolarization through the atria, and resultant contraction

QRS complex

- Appearance—includes Q, R, and S waves
- Represents—contraction of the ventricles; the QRS complex is larger than the P wave because the ventricles are larger and produce a larger electrical impulse than the atria

Q wave

- Appearance—downward deflection
- Represents—an impulse traveling down the septum toward the Purkinje fibers

R wave

- Appearance—large, upward spike
- Represents—an impulse going through the left ventricle

S wave

- Appearance—downward deflection
- Represents—an impulse going through both ventricles

T wave

- Appearance—upward curve
- Represents—recovery of the ventricles

U wave

- Appearance—small, upward curve sometimes found after the T wave
- Represents—may be seen in normal individuals, in patients who experience slow recovery of Purkinje fibers, or in patients who have low potassium levels or other metabolic disturbances

P-R interval

- Appearance—starts at the beginning of the P wave and ends at the beginning of the next R wave
- Represents—the time it takes for an electrical impulse to travel from the SA node to the AV node

Q-T interval

- Appearance—includes the QRS complex, S-T segment, and T wave
- Represents—the time it takes for the ventricles to contract and recover

S-T segment

- Appearance—connects the end of the QRS complex with the beginning of the T wave
- Represents—the time between contraction of ventricles and recovery

Emergencies

Assisting in a Disaster

Type of Disaster	Action to Take
Weather disaster, such as a flood or hurricane	• Report to the community command post. • Have your credentials with you. • Receive an identifying tag or vest and assignment. • Accept only an assignment that is appropriate for your abilities. • Expect to be part of a team. • Document what medical care each victim receives on his or her disaster tag.
Office fire	• Activate the alarm system. • Use a fire extinguisher if the fire is confined to a small container, such as a trash can. • Turn off oxygen. • Shut windows and doors. • Seal doors with wet cloths to prevent smoke from entering. • If evacuation is necessary, proceed quietly and calmly. Direct ambulatory patients and family members to the appropriate exit route. Assist patients who need help leaving the building.

Type of Disaster	Action to Take
Bioterrorist attack	• Be alert for rapidly increasing incidence of disease in a healthy population (clusters).
	• Take appropriate isolation precautions.
	• Use standard precautions when cleaning/decontaminating patient rooms and equipment.
	• Inform local health departments of suspected bioterrorism agent.
Chemical emergency	• Don appropriate PPE to avoid secondary contamination.
	• Identify the chemical if possible and report to the local authorities.
	• Determine if there is a protocol for the specific chemical, if known.
	• Assist with patient decontamination.
	• Monitor patient's CABs and vital signs if indicated.
	• Document what medical care each victim receives.
	• Arrange for patient transport if necessary.
Mass casualties	• Assess the situation for safety.
	• If there is an explosion, do not go toward the explosion.
	• Report to the community command post.
	• Triage victims as necessary.
	• Render first aid as required.
	• Document what medical care each victim receives.

continued

Type of Disaster	Action to Take
Radiation emergencies	• Assess for contamination (contact with radioisotope released in liquid or powder form) or exposure from an external source (for example, from a nuclear power plant accident).
	• If victim is contaminated, use PPE appropriate for radiation protection, assess for amount of contamination, and decontaminate victim following approved decontamination procedures.
	• If victim is exposed, look for signs of acute radiation syndrome (ARS) and assist physician in management of multisystem ARS symptoms.

Basic Life Support: Key Components

Component	Recommendations		
	Adults	Children	Infants
Recognition	Unresponsive, all ages		
	No breathing or abnormal breathing, such as gasping		
	No pulse palpated within 10 seconds (healthcare professionals)		
CPR sequence	CAB	CAB	CAB
Compression rate	At least 100/min		
Compression depth	At least 2 inches	2 inches or 1/3 anteroposterior chest circumference	1½ inches or 1/3 anteroposterior chest circumference
Chest wall recoil	Complete recoil between compressions		
Compression interruptions	Limit chest compression interruptions to less than 10 seconds, if at all		
Airway	Head tilt–chin lift		Healthcare professionals only—jaw thrust if indicated by trauma
Compression-to-ventilation ratio	30:2 (1 or 2 rescuers)	30:2 (Single rescuer) 15:2 (Two healthcare professional rescuers)	30:2 (Single rescuer) 15:2 (Two healthcare professional rescuers)
Ventilations for untrained rescuer	Compressions only		
Defibrillation	• Use AED as soon as possible. • Minimize interruptions in chest compressions before and after shock. • Resume compressions immediately after each shock.		

Source: Adapted from 2010 American Heart Association Guidelines for Cardiopulmonary Resuscitation and Emergency Cardiovascular Care Service, Part 4, Table 1.

Calling Poison Control (800-222-1222)

Information you will need to know:

- The patient's age
- The name of the poison
- The amount of poison swallowed
- When the poison was swallowed
- Whether or not the person has vomited
- How long it will take to get the patient to a medical facility

Caring for a Patient Who Is Vomiting

CRITICAL PROCEDURE STEPS

1. Wash your hands and put on exam gloves and other PPE.
2. Ask the patient when and how the vomiting started and how frequently it occurs. Find out whether she is nauseated or in pain.
3. Give the patient an emesis basin to collect vomit. Observe and document its amount, color, odor, and consistency. Particularly note blood, bile, undigested food, or feces in the vomit.
4. Place a cool compress on the patient's forehead to make her more comfortable. Offer water and paper tissues or a towel to clean her mouth.
5. Monitor for signs of dehydration, such as confusion, irritability, and flushed, dry skin. Also monitor for signs of electrolyte imbalances, such as leg cramps or an irregular pulse.

6. If requested, assist by laying out supplies and equipment for the physician to use in administering intravenous fluids and electrolytes. Administer an antinausea drug if prescribed.
7. Prepare the patient for diagnostic tests if instructed.
8. Remove the gloves and wash your hands.

Cast Care

- Report any of the following to the physician immediately: pain, swelling, discoloration of exposed portions, lack of pulsation and warmth, or the inability to move exposed parts.
- Keep the casted extremity elevated for the first day.
- Avoid indenting the cast until it is completely dry.
- Check the movement and sensation of the visible extremities frequently.
- Restrict strenuous activities for the first few days.
- Avoid allowing the affected limb to hang down for any length of time.
- Do not put anything inside the cast.
- Keep the cast dry.
- Follow the physician's orders about restricting activities.

Choosing PPE During an Emergency

Equipment	Conditions for Use
Gloves	Chance of contact with blood or other body secretion or excretion during emergency

continued

Equipment	Conditions for Use
Goggles and mask or face shield and possibly head cover	Chance of blood or other body secretion or excretion being splattered, coughed, or sprayed onto the mucous membranes of the eyes, mouth, or nose
Gown and possibly booties	Chance of contact with excessive bleeding or secretion and excretion
Pocket mask or mouth shield	Needed for CPR or rescue breathing

Cleaning Minor Wounds

CRITICAL PROCEDURE STEPS

1. Wash your hands and put on gloves.
2. Dip gauze squares in warm, soapy water.
3. Wash the wound from the center outward, using a new gauze square for each cleansing motion.
4. Remove debris as you wash.
5. Rinse the wound.
6. Pat the wound dry with sterile gauze.
7. Cover the wound with a dry, sterile dressing.
8. Bandage the dressing in place.
9. Properly dispose of contaminated materials.
10. Remove gloves and wash your hands.
11. Instruct the patient on wound care.
12. Document the procedure in the patient's chart.

Concussion

PATIENT EDUCATION TIPS

After a concussion, teach patients the following guidelines:

- Inform the patient that the first 24 hours after the injury are the most critical.

- Tell the patient to refrain from strenuous activity, to rest, and to return to regular activity gradually. Instruct the patient to avoid using pain medicines other than acetaminophen, unless the drugs are approved by the physician.

- Advise the patient to eat lightly, especially if nausea and vomiting occur.

- Tell a family member to check on the patient every few hours. The family member should make sure the patient knows his own name, his location, and the name of the family member.

- Instruct the family member to call for medical assistance immediately if the patient exhibits any of these warning signs:
  - Any symptom that is getting worse, such as head-aches, sleepiness, or nausea, including nausea that doesn't go away
  - Changes in behavior, such as irritability or confusion
  - Dilated pupils (pupils that are bigger than normal) or pupils of different sizes
  - Trouble walking or speaking
  - Drainage of bloody or clear fluids from ears or nose
  - Vomiting
  - Seizures

continued

- Weakness or numbness in the arms or legs
- A less serious head injury in a patient taking blood thinners or who has a bleeding disorder such as hemophilia

Controlling Bleeding

CRITICAL PROCEDURE STEPS

1. If you have time, wash your hands and put on exam gloves, face protection, and a gown.
2. Using a clean or sterile dressing, apply direct pressure over the wound.
3. If blood soaks through the dressing, do not remove it. Apply an additional dressing over the original one.
4. If possible, elevate the body part that is bleeding.
5. If direct pressure and elevation do not stop the bleeding, apply pressure over the nearest pressure point between the bleeding and the heart. For example, if the wound is on the lower arm, apply pressure on the brachial artery. For a lower-leg wound, apply pressure on the femoral artery in the groin.
6. When the doctor or EMT arrives, assist as requested.
7. After the patient has been transferred to a hospital, properly dispose of contaminated materials.
8. Remove the gloves and wash your hands.
9. Document your care in the patient's chart.

Estimating the Extent of a Burn

Use these charts to calculate the percentage of body surface affected by burns.

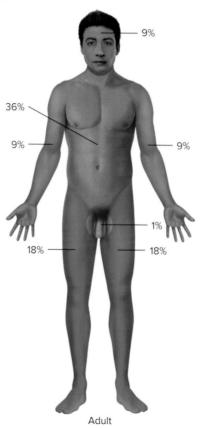

9%

36%

9%

9%

1%

18%

18%

Adult

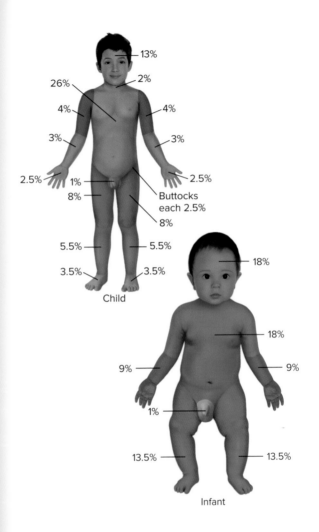

13%

2%

26%

4%   4%

3%   3%

2.5%   2.5%

1%

8%   Buttocks
         each 2.5%

         8%

5.5%   5.5%

3.5%   3.5%

Child

18%

18%

9%   9%

1%

13.5%   13.5%

Infant

Fractures, Dislocations, Sprains, and Strains

Basic emergency steps

- Keep the person calm and limit his movement.
- Assess him for any other injuries.
- Notify the doctor or call EMS. Do not move the patient until the doctor or EMS arrives.
- If the skin is broken, cover with a sterile dressing.
- Immobilize the extremity with a splint or sling. Use rolled-up newspaper, strips of wood, etc., to immobilize above and below the injury.
- Do not try to put the bone back into place. Immobilize it in the position in which it was found.
- Place an ice pack on the affected area.
- Monitor him for signs of shock.
- Assess for signs of lack of circulation.

Performing an Emergency Assessment

CRITICAL PROCEDURE STEPS

1. Put on gloves.
2. Form a general impression of the patient.
3. Gather information from the patient or bystanders about the incident.
4. Assess an unresponsive patient by tapping her shoulder and asking "Are you OK?"
5. Assess the patient's circulation, airway, and breathing. Perform CPR as needed.
6. Perform a head-to-toe focused exam.
7. Recheck vital signs and assess for signs of shock.

continued

8. Report your findings to the doctor or EMS.
9. Document your findings in the patient chart.
10. Assist the doctor or EMS as requested.
11. Dispose of hazardous waste as required.
12. Remove your gloves and wash your hands.

Eye Irrigation

CRITICAL PROCEDURE STEPS

1. Identify the patient and explain the procedure.
2. Review the physician's order.
3. Compare the solution with the order three times.
4. Wash your hands and put on gloves, a gown, and a face shield.
5. Assemble the supplies.
6. Ask the patient to lie down or sit with his head tilted back and to the side that is being irrigated.
7. Place a towel over the patient's shoulder and have the patient hold the basin under the eye that is being irrigated.
8. Pour the solution into a sterile basin.
9. Fill the irrigating syringe with solution.
10. Hold a tissue on the patient's cheekbone with your nondominant hand, and press down to expose the patient's eye socket.
11. Holding the tip of the syringe ½ inch from the eye, direct the solution onto the patient's conjunctiva from the inside to the outside.

12. Do not allow the solution to enter the other eye.

13. Do not direct the solution toward the cornea.

14. Do not use excessive force.

15. Refill the syringe and continue the irrigation until the prescribed amount of solution is used.

16. Dry the area around the eye with tissues.

17. Properly dispose of disposable supplies.

18. Remove your gloves, gown, and face shield, and wash your hands.

19. Record in the patient's chart the procedure, the amount of solution used, the time of administration, and the eye(s) irrigated.

20. Put on gloves and clean the equipment and room according to OSHA guidelines.

Gynecology

Assisting with a Gynecology Exam

CRITICAL PROCEDURE STEPS

1. Gather equipment and make sure all items are in working order. Correctly label the slide and/or the collection vials.

2. Identify the patient and explain the procedure.

3. Have the patient remove all clothing, including underwear, and put the gown on with the opening in the front.

continued

4. Ask the patient to sit on the edge of the examining table with the drape until the licensed practitioner arrives.

5. When the licensed practitioner is ready, have the patient place her feet in the stirrups and move her buttocks to the edge of the table.

6. Provide the physician with gloves and an exam lamp as she examines the genitalia by inspection and palpation.

7. Pass the speculum to the licensed practitioner. To increase patient comfort, you may place it in warm water before handing it to the practitioner. Do not use a water-based lubricant.

8. For the Pap (Papanicolaou) smear, be prepared to pass a cotton-tipped applicator and cervical brush, broom, or scraper for the collection of the specimens.

9. Have the labeled slide or vial available for the licensed practitioner.

10. Once the specimen is on the slide, a cytology fixative must be applied immediately. A spray fixative is common, and it should be held 6 inches from the slide and sprayed lightly with a back-and-forth motion. Allow the slide to dry completely.

11. Cells collected for thin-layer preparation should be washed into the collection vial.

12. After the licensed practitioner removes the speculum, provide the practitioner with additional lubricant as needed for the digital exam.

13. Upon completion of the exam, help the patient into a supine or sitting position.

14. Provide tissues or moist wipes for the patient to remove the lubricant, and ask the patient to get dressed.

15. Explain the procedure for communicating the laboratory results.

16. After the patient has left, don gloves and clean the exam room and equipment.

17. Dispose of the disposable speculum, specimen collection devices, and other contaminated waste in a biohazardous waste container.

18. Store the supplies, straighten the room, and discard the used exam paper on the table.

19. Prepare the laboratory requisition slip, and place it and the specimen in the proper place for transport to an outside laboratory.

20. Remove your gloves and wash your hands.

21. Document the specimen and complete the laboratory log if needed.

Assisting with a Cervical Biopsy

CRITICAL PROCEDURE STEPS

1. Identify the patient and introduce yourself.

2. Look at the patient's chart and ask the patient to confirm information or explain any changes. Specific patient information you need to ask about and note in the chart includes the following:

continued

- Date of birth and Social Security number (verify that you have the correct chart for the correct patient)
- Date of last menstrual period
- Method of contraception, if any
- Previous gynecologic surgery
- Use of hormone replacement therapy or other steroids

3. Describe the biopsy procedure to the patient, noting that a piece of tissue will be removed to diagnose the cause of her problem. Explain that it may be painful but only for the brief moment during which tissue is taken.

4. Give the patient a gown, if needed, and a drape. Direct her to undress from the waist down and to wrap the drape around herself. Tell her to sit at the end of the examining table.

5. Wash your hands and put on exam gloves.

6. Using sterile method, open the sterile pack to create a sterile field on the tray or Mayo stand, and arrange the instruments with transfer forceps. Add the vaginal speculum and sterile supplies to the sterile field.

7. When the licensed practitioner arrives in the examining room, ask the patient to lie back, place her heels in the stirrups of the table, and move her buttocks to the edge of the table.

8. Assist the licensed practitioner by arranging the drape so that only the genitalia are exposed, and place the light so that the genitalia are illuminated.

9. Use transfer forceps to hand instruments and supplies to the licensed practitioner as he

requests them. You may don sterile gloves and hand the practitioner supplies and instruments directly. When he is ready to obtain the biopsy, tell the patient that it may hurt. If she seems particularly fearful, instruct her to take a deep breath and let it out slowly.

10. When the licensed practitioner hands you the instrument with the tissue specimen, place the specimen in the specimen container and discard the instrument in the appropriate container.

11. Label the specimen container with the patient's name, the date and time, cervical or endocervical (as indicated by the licensed practitioner), the practitioner's name, and your initials.

12. Place the container and the cytology laboratory requisition form in the envelope or bag provided by the laboratory.

13. When the practitioner has removed the vaginal speculum, properly clean instruments as needed and dispose of used supplies and disposable instruments.

14. Remove the gloves and wash your hands.

15. Tell the patient that she may get dressed. Inform her that she may have some vaginal bleeding for a couple of days, and provide her with a sanitary napkin. Instruct her not to take tub baths or have intercourse and not to use tampons for 2 days. Encourage her to call the office if she experiences problems or has questions.

16. Document the procedure as appropriate.

Cervical Specimen Collection and Submission Guidelines

In order to ensure that the cervical specimen collected is adequate for optimal screening, the American Society of Cytopathology has certain clinical guidelines. As a medical assistant, you will be responsible for helping the physician implement these guidelines.

Collecting patient information:

- Scheduling a patient appointment about 2 weeks after the patient's last menstrual period
- Instructing patients not to douche; use tampons, foams, or jellies; or have sexual intercourse 48 hours prior to the test
- Completing a lab requisition form, which includes the following information:
  - Patient name (note any recent name changes)
  - Date of birth
  - Menstrual status (last menstrual period, hysterectomy, etc.)
  - Any patient risk factors
  - Specimen source

Completing a specimen label:

- Glass slide
  - Label the frosted end of the slide with the patient's first and last name
  - Include an additional identifier, such as the patient record number
- Liquid samples
  - Complete all requested information on the label and affix to the vial

Assisting During the Exam of a Pregnant Patient

CRITICAL PROCEDURE STEPS

Providing Patient Information

1. Identify the patient and introduce yourself.
2. Assess the patient's need for education by asking appropriate questions.
3. Provide any appropriate instructions or materials.
4. Ask the patient whether she has any special concerns or questions about her pregnancy that she might want to discuss with the licensed practitioner.
5. Communicate the patient's concerns or questions to the licensed practitioner; include all pertinent background information on the patient.

Ensuring Comfort During the Exam

1. Identify the patient and introduce yourself.
2. Wash your hands.
3. Explain the procedure to the patient.
4. Provide a gown or drape, and instruct the patient in the proper way to wear it after disrobing. (Allow the patient privacy while disrobing, and assist only if she requests help.)
5. Ask the patient to step on the stool or the pullout step of the examining table.
6. Assist the patient onto the examining table.
7. Keeping position restrictions in mind, help the patient into the position requested by the physician.
8. Provide and adjust additional drapes as needed.

continued

9. Keep in mind any difficulties the patient may have in achieving a certain position; suggest alternative positions whenever possible.

10. Minimize the time the patient must spend in uncomfortable positions.

11. If the patient appears to be uncomfortable during the procedure, ask whether she would like to reposition herself or take a break; assist as necessary.

12. To prevent pelvic pooling of blood and subsequent dizziness or hyperventilation, allow the patient time to adjust to sitting before standing after she has been lying on the examining table.

Pap Smear Classifications

Understanding Pap Smear Results

Classification	What It Means	Tests and Treatments That May Be Indicated
Unsatisfactory	Inadequate sampling or other interfering substance	The test must be repeated.
Negative	Cells appear normal and no identifiable infection is evident.	Continue routine Pap smears.
Benign	Noncancerous cells, but smear shows infection, irritation, or normal cell repair	Continue routine Pap smears.
Atypical cells of uncertain significance: either ASC-US or ASC-H	Abnormal cells are present, but it is uncertain what these cells may indicate.	Repeat the Pap smear; sometimes changes can go away without treatment. Estrogen cream for women who are at or near menopause Follow-up test of cells for presence of high-risk HPV (human papillomavirus). If HPV is present, a colposcopy is performed.

continued

Classification	What It Means	Tests and Treatments That May Be Indicated
Low-grade changes (mild dysplasia)	Cells have changes that are not cancer but have the potential to be cancer. Cell changes may be caused by HPV infection.	HPV testing; repeat Pap test; colposcopy. If abnormal tissue is found, then endocervical curettage or biopsy.
High-grade changes (moderate to severe dysplasia or carcinoma in situ, depending upon amount and location of cells)	Cells have more evident changes and look very different than normal cells.	Colposcopy and biopsy; LEEP procedure, cryotherapy, laser therapy, or conization
Squamous cell carcinoma	Cells invade deep into the cervix and other tissues or organs.	Immediate treatment, including surgical removal; rare finding in well-screened populations such as the United States

Source: Based on the Bethesda System for Classification of Papanicolaou Smear.

Heat and Cold Therapy Guidelines

Administering Cryotherapy

CRITICAL PROCEDURE STEPS

1. Check the physician's order for location and length of time of therapy.
2. Identify the patient and explain the procedure.
3. Have the patient undress and put on a gown if required.
4. Wash your hands and put on gloves.
5. Position the patient comfortably and drape appropriately.
6. Prepare the therapy as ordered.
7. Place the device on the patient's affected body part.
8. Ask the patient how the device feels.
9. Leave in place for the ordered amount of time (no longer than 20 minutes).
10. Remove the application and observe the area for reduced swelling, redness, and pain.
11. If the patient has a dressing, replace it.
12. Assist the patient as necessary.
13. Remove any equipment and supplies and properly dispose of used disposable materials.
14. Remove your gloves and wash your hands.
15. Document the treatment and your observations in the patient chart.

Administering Thermotherapy

CRITICAL PROCEDURE STEPS

1. Check the physician's order for location and length of time of therapy.
2. Identify the patient and explain the procedure.
3. Have the patient undress and put on a gown if required.
4. Wash your hands and put on gloves.
5. Position the patient comfortably and drape appropriately.
6. If the patient has a dressing, check the dressing for blood and change if necessary.
7. Prepare the therapy as ordered.
8. Check the temperature by touch and assess the patient for signs of adverse skin conditions.
9. Place the device on the patient's affected body part.
10. Ask the patient how the device feels.
11. Leave in place for the ordered amount of time.
12. Check periodically for signs of adverse skin conditions.
13. Remove the application and observe the area.
14. Replace the patient's dressing if indicated.
15. Help the patient dress, if necessary.
16. Remove any equipment and supplies and properly dispose of used disposable materials.
17. Remove your gloves and wash your hands.
18. Document the treatment and your observations in the patient chart.

Contraindications to Heat and Cold Therapy

Therapy	Contraindications
Dry and moist cold applications	Severe circulatory problems, inability to tolerate weight of device, pain caused by application (more common with moist cold)
Dry and moist hot applications	Possibility of hemorrhage, malignancy; acute inflammation, such as appendicitis; severe circulation problems; pain caused by weight of device

Holter Monitor

CRITICAL PROCEDURE STEPS

1. Identify the patient and explain the procedure.
2. Have the patient remove clothing from the waist up.
3. Place the patient in a comfortable position.
4. Prepare the patient's skin at the electrode sites.
5. Apply the electrodes.
6. Attach the patient cable.
7. Attach the wires to the electrodes.
8. Insert a fresh battery and position the unit.
9. Tape wires, cable, and electrodes as necessary.
10. Insert a microchip or cassette and turn on the unit.
11. Ensure that the unit is on and note the start time in the patient's chart.

continued

12. Instruct the patient on proper use of the monitor and how to make entries in the diary.
13. Schedule the patient's return visit.
14. On the patient's return visit, remove the electrodes and clean the electrode sites.
15. Wash your hands.
16. Transfer the data from the monitor to the patient's chart.
17. Document all parts of the procedure.

PATIENT EDUCATION TIPS

Before Holter monitoring, instruct the patient to

- Continue normal activities during Holter monitoring.
- Record all activities, emotional upsets, physical symptoms, and medications taken.
- Wear loose-fitting clothing that opens in the front.
- Avoid magnets, metal detectors, high-voltage areas, and electric blankets during the monitoring period.
- Avoid getting the monitor wet.
- Check the monitor to make sure it is working.

Immunization* Schedule

2015 Recommended Immunizations for Children from 7 Through 18 Years Old

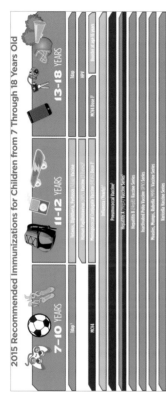

7–10 YEARS
- Tdap[1]
- MCV4[3]

11–12 YEARS
- Tetanus, Diphtheria, Pertussis (Tdap) Vaccine[1]
- Meningococcal Conjugate Vaccine (MCV4) Dose 1[3]
- Human Papillomavirus (HPV)[2]
- Pneumococcal Vaccine[5]
- Hepatitis A (HepA) Vaccine Series[6]
- Hepatitis B (HepB) Vaccine Series
- Inactivated Polio Vaccine (IPV) Series
- Measles, Mumps, Rubella (MMR) Vaccine Series
- Varicella Vaccine Series

13–18 YEARS
- Tdap
- HPV
- MCV4 Dose 2[3]
- Booster at age 16 years

These shaded boxes indicate when the vaccine is recommended for all children unless your doctor tells you that your child cannot safely receive the vaccine.

These shaded boxes indicate the vaccine should be given if a child is catching-up on missed vaccines.

These shaded boxes indicate the vaccine is recommended for children with certain health conditions that put them at high risk for serious diseases. Note that healthy children can get the HepA series! See vaccine-specific recommendations at www.cdc.gov/vaccines/pubs/ACIP-list.htm.

FOOTNOTES

[1] Tdap vaccine is recommended at age 11 or 12 to protect against tetanus, diphtheria and pertussis. If your child has not received any or all of the DTaP vaccine series, or if you don't know if your child has received these shots, your child needs a single dose of Tdap when they are 7–10 years old. Talk to your child's health care provider to find out if they need additional catch-up vaccines.

[2] All 11 or 12 year olds – both girls and boys – should receive 3 doses of HPV vaccine to protect against HPV-related disease. The full HPV vaccine series should be given as recommended for best protection.

[3] Meningococcal conjugate vaccine (MCV) is recommended at age 11 or 12. A booster shot is recommended at age 16. Teens who received MCV for the first time at age 13 through 15 years will need a one-time booster dose between the ages of 16 and 18 years. If your teenager missed getting the vaccine altogether, ask their health care provider about getting it now, especially if your teenager is about to move into a college dorm or military barracks.

[4] Everyone 6 months of age and older—including preteens and teens—should get a flu vaccine every year. Children under the age of 9 years may require more than one dose. Talk to your child's health care provider to find out if they need more than one dose.

[5] Pneumococcal Conjugate Vaccine (PCV13) and Pneumococcal Polysaccharide Vaccine (PPSV23) are recommended for some children 6 through 18 years old with certain medical conditions that place them at high risk. Talk to your healthcare provider about pneumococcal vaccines and what factors may place your child at high risk for pneumococcal disease.

[6] Hepatitis A vaccination is recommended for older children with certain medical conditions that place them at high risk. HepA vaccine is licensed, safe, and effective for all children of all ages. Even if your child is not at high risk, you may decide you want your child protected against HepA. Talk to your healthcare provider about HepA vaccine and what factors may place your child at high risk for HepA.

For more information, call toll free 1-800-CDC-INFO (1-800-232-4636) or visit http://www.cdc.gov/vaccines/teens

U.S. Department of
Health and Human Services
Centers for Disease
Control and Prevention

CDC

American Academy
of Pediatrics
DEDICATED TO THE HEALTH OF ALL CHILDREN™

AMERICAN ACADEMY OF
FAMILY PHYSICIANS
STRONG MEDICINE FOR AMERICA

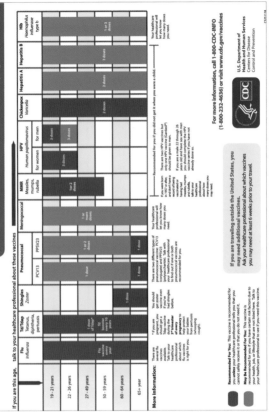

84

2015 Recommended Immunizations for Children from Birth Through 6 Years Old

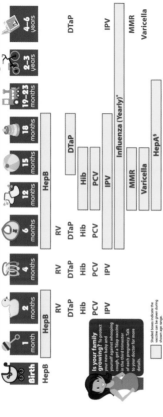

	Birth	1 month	2 months	4 months	6 months		12 months	15 months	18 months	19–23 months	2–3 years	4–6 years
HepB	HepB	HepB			HepB							
RV			RV	RV	RV							
DTaP			DTaP	DTaP	DTaP			DTaP				DTaP
Hib			Hib	Hib	Hib		Hib					
PCV			PCV	PCV	PCV		PCV					
IPV			IPV	IPV		IPV						IPV
Influenza						Influenza (Yearly)*						
MMR							MMR					MMR
Varicella							Varicella					Varicella
HepA							HepA§					

Shaded boxes indicate the vaccine can be given during shown age range.

Is your family growing? To protect your new baby and yourself against whooping cough, get a Tdap vaccine in the third trimester of each pregnancy. Talk to your doctor for more details.

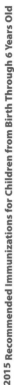

NOTE: If your child misses a shot, you don't need to start over, just go back to your child's doctor for the next shot. Talk with your child's doctor if you have questions about vaccines.

FOOTNOTES:
* Two doses given at least four weeks apart are recommended for children aged 6 months through 8 years of age who are getting an influenza (flu) vaccine for the first time and for some other children in this age group.

§ Two doses of HepA vaccine are needed for lasting protection. The first dose of HepA vaccine should be given between 12 months and 23 months of age. The second dose should be given 6 to 18 months later. HepA vaccination may be given to any child 12 months and older to protect against HepA. Children and adolescents who did not receive the HepA vaccine and are at high-risk, should be vaccinated against HepA.

If your child has any medical conditions that put him at risk for infection or is traveling outside the United States, talk to your child's doctor about additional vaccines that he may need.

For more information, call toll free
1-800-CDC-INFO (1-800-232-4636)
or visit
http://www.cdc.gov/vaccines

U.S. Department of Health and Human Services
Centers for Disease Control and Prevention

AMERICAN ACADEMY OF FAMILY PHYSICIANS
STRONG MEDICINE FOR AMERICA

SEE BACK PAGE FOR MORE INFORMATION ON VACCINE-PREVENTABLE DISEASES AND THE VACCINES THAT PREVENT THEM.

American Academy of Pediatrics
DEDICATED TO THE HEALTH OF ALL CHILDREN™

Medication Administration

Rights of Drug Administration

Basic Rights

1. **Right patient**—always check the patient's name and date of birth.

2. **Right drug**—compare the name of the prescribed drug in the patient's chart with the drug container label. Check three times!

3. **Right dose**—compare the dose ordered with the dose you prepare.

4. **Right route**—make sure the administration route you have prepared matches the prescribed route.

5. **Right time**—give the drug at the prescribed time.

6. **Right documentation**—document immediately after administering the drug.

Additional Rights

7. **Right reason**—the patient and person administering the medication should know the reason for the medication.

8. **Right to know**—the patient should be informed of the reason, the effects, and the side effects of a medication.

9. **Right to refuse**—the authorized prescriber should be informed and the refusal should be documented.

10. **Right technique**—use the proper administration technique.

A violation of any of these rights constitutes a medication error.

Triple Check

Perform a triple check by checking the medication three times before administering. Check the medication three times even if the dose is prepackaged, labeled, and ready to be administered.

1. **1st check**—when you take the medication from the storage container and match it to the medication administration record (MAR)
2. **2nd check**—when you prepare the medication
3. **3rd check**—before you close the storage container or just before you administer the medication to the patient

Types of Drug Administration

Administering buccal or sublingual drugs

CRITICAL PROCEDURE STEPS

1. Identify the patient and wash your hands.
2. Select the ordered drug.
3. Check the medication rights.
4. If you are unfamiliar with the drug, check the PDR®, read the package insert, or speak with the licensed practitioner.
5. Ask the patient about drug or food allergies.
6. Perform calculations needed to provide the prescribed dose.

continued

7. Open the container and tap the correct number into the cap.

8. Tap the tablets or capsules into a paper cup.

9. Recap the container immediately.

10. Tell the patient not to chew or swallow.

11. *Buccal*—place the medication between the cheek and the gum until it dissolves.

    Sublingual—place the medication under the tongue until it dissolves.

12. Instruct the patient not to eat, drink, or smoke until the tablet is completely dissolved.

13. Remain with the patient until the tablet dissolves.

14. Wash your hands.

15. Give the patient written and oral information about the drug and answer any questions.

16. Document the date, time, drug name, dosage, expiration date, lot number, manufacturer, route, site, significant patient reactions, and patient education in the chart.

Administering eardrops

CRITICAL PROCEDURE STEPS

1. Identify the patient and explain the procedure.

2. Review the medication order.

3. Compare the drug with the medication order three times.

4. Ask the patient about drug allergies.

5. Wash your hands and put on gloves.
6. Assemble the supplies.
7. Warm the medication.
8. Have the patient lie on her side with the affected ear up.
9. Straighten the ear canal by pulling upward and outward for adults or down and back for infants and children.
10. Hold the dropper ½ inch from the ear canal.
11. Gently squeeze the dropper or bottle to administer the ordered number of drops.
12. Have the patient remain in this position for 10 minutes.
13. If ordered, loosely place a small cotton ball in the patient's ear.
14. Observe for adverse reactions.
15. Repeat the procedure for the other ear if indicated.
16. Instruct the patient on how to administer the drops at home.
17. Provide written instructions.
18. Remove the cotton after 15 minutes.
19. Properly dispose of disposable supplies.
20. Remove the gloves and wash your hands.
21. Document the date, time, drug name, number of drops, drug concentration, route, site, significant patient reactions, and patient education in the chart.

CRITICAL PROCEDURE STEPS

1. Identify the patient and explain the procedure.
2. Review the medication order.
3. Compare the drug with the medication order three times.
4. Ask the patient about drug allergies.
5. Wash your hands and put on gloves.
6. Assemble the supplies.
7. Ask the patient to lie down or sit with her head tilted back.
8. Give the patient a tissue to blot excess medication as needed.
9. Remove an eye patch, if present.
10. Ask the patient to look at the ceiling and keep both eyes open during the procedure.
11. With a tissue, gently pull the lower eyelid down, creating a pocket.

Eyedrops

12. Rest your dominant hand on the patient's forehead, holding the filled eyedropper or bottle ½ inch from the conjunctiva.
13. Drop the prescribed number of drops into the pocket.

Creams or Ointments

12. Rest your dominant hand on the patient's forehead, holding the tube or applicator above the conjunctiva.

13. Without touching the eyelid or conjunctiva with the applicator, apply a thin ribbon of cream or ointment along the inside edge of the lower eyelid, working from the inner to the outer side.

All Medications

14. Release the lower lid and instruct the patient to gently close her eyes.
15. Repeat the procedure for the other eye if indicated.
16. Remove any excess medication by wiping each eyelid with a tissue from the inner to the outer side.
17. Apply a clean eye patch if necessary.
18. Ask if the patient felt any discomfort and observe for adverse reactions.
19. Instruct the patient on self-administration of medication and patch application as necessary.
20. Ask the patient to repeat the instructions.
21. Provide written instructions.
22. Properly dispose of disposable supplies.
23. Remove the gloves and wash your hands.
24. Document the date, time, drug name, number of drops, drug concentration, route, site, significant patient reactions, and patient education in the chart.

CRITICAL PROCEDURE STEPS

1. Identify the patient and wash your hands.
2. Select the ordered drug.
3. Check the medication rights.
4. If you are unfamiliar with the drug, check the PDR®, read the package insert, or speak with the physician.
5. Ask the patient about drug or food allergies.
6. Perform calculations needed to provide the prescribed dose.

Tablets or Capsules

7. Open the container and tap the correct number into the cap.
8. Tap the tablets or capsules into a paper cup.
9. Recap the container immediately.
10. Give the patient the cup and a glass of water or juice.

Liquid

7. Shake a liquid suspension.
8. Locate the correct mark on the medicine cup and pour in the correct amount of medication. Place your palm over the label so that the medication does not run onto the label.
9. After pouring the drug, place the cup on a flat surface and recheck the level.
10. Give the medicine cup to the patient and have the patient drink it.

After Administering the Drug

11. Wash your hands.

12. Give the patient written and oral information about the drug and answer any questions.

13. Document the date, time, drug name, dosage, expiration date, lot number, manufacturer, route, site, significant patient reactions, and patient education in the chart.

Administering and removing transdermal medications

CRITICAL PROCEDURE STEPS

1. Identify the patient, wash your hands, and put on gloves.

2. Select the ordered transdermal patch.

3. Check the medication rights.

4. If you are unfamiliar with the drug, check the PDR®, read the package insert, or speak with the physician.

5. Perform calculations needed to provide the prescribed dose.

6. Ask the patient about any drug allergies.

Applying the Patch

7. Remove the patch from its pouch and peel off the plastic backing.

8. Demonstrate to the patient how to remove the plastic backing.

9. Apply the patch to a reasonably hair-free site.

continued

10. Instruct the patient how to apply the patch.

11. Avoid using extremities below the knee or elbow, skin folds, scar tissue, or burned areas.

Removing the Patch

12. Gently lift and slowly peel the patch back from the skin.

13. Wash the area with soap and dry it with a towel.

14. Explain to the patient that the area may be warm and red but that the redness will disappear.

15. Apply lotion to the area if it feels dry.

16. Instruct the patient to advise the physician if the redness doesn't go away or if a rash appears.

17. Never apply a patch to a site that was just used.

After Applying or Removing the Patch

18. Wash your hands and instruct the patient to do so after applying or removing a patch.

19. Give the patient written and oral information about the drug and answer any questions.

20. Document the date, time, drug name, dosage, expiration date, lot number, manufacturer, route, site, significant patient reactions, and patient education in the chart.

Suggested Needle Gauge, Length, Injection Amount, and Location

Age	Needle Size	Needle Length	Maximum Injection Amount	Location
		Intradermal (ID)		
All ages	25 to 26 gauge	⅜ to ½ inch	0.1 mL	Interior aspect of forearm (most common)
		Subcutaneous (subcut)		
1 to 12 months	23 to 27 gauge	⅝ inch	1 mL	Fatty tissue over anterior lateral thigh muscle
>12 months to adults	23 to 27 gauge	½ to ¾ inch; ⅝ inch most common	1 mL	Fatty tissue over anterior lateral thigh muscle or over triceps

continued

Intramuscular (IM)			
1 to 28 days	18 to 23 gauge	⅝ inch	1 mL	Anterolateral thigh muscle
1 to 12 months	18 to 23 gauge	1 inch	1 mL	Anterolateral thigh muscle
1 to 2 years	18 to 23 gauge	1 to 1¼ inch ⅝ to 1 inch	1 mL	Anterolateral thigh muscle Deltoid muscle of arm
3 to 18 years	18 to 23 gauge	⅝ to 1 inch 1 to 1¼ inch	2 mL	Deltoid muscle of arm Anterolateral thigh muscle
All adults ≥19 years <130 lb	18 to 23 gauge	⅝ to 1 inch	3 mL	Deltoid muscle of arm
Adults ≥19 years Female 130 to 200 lb; male 130 to 260 lb	18 to 23 gauge	1 to 1½ inch	3 mL	Deltoid muscle of arm
Adults ≥19 years Female 200+ lb; male 260+ lb	18 to 23 gauge	1½ inch	3 mL	Deltoid muscle of arm

Syringes

Choose the correct syringe based on the type of medication and the volume administered.

1 mL
tuberculin

3 mL
standard syringe

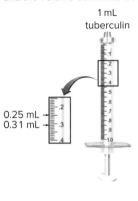

0.25 mL →
0.31 mL →

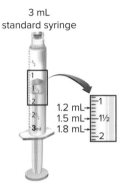

1.2 mL →
1.5 mL →
1.8 mL →

50 unit Lo-Dose
syringe

Standard 100 unit
syringe

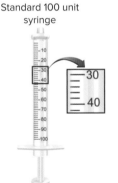

Each large mark indicates 5 units.	Each large mark indicates 10 units.
Each small mark indicates 1 unit.	Each small mark indicates 2 units.

Conversion Charts for Measurements

Metric to apothecary and standard (household)

Volume

- 5 mL = 1 teaspoon
- 15 mL = 1 tablespoon
- 30 mL = 1 fluid ounce
- 500 mL = 1 pint
- 1,000 mL = 1 quart

Weight

- 0.06 g = 1 grain
- 0.5 g = 7¾ gr
- 1 g = 15 gr
- 4 g = 1 dram
- 30 g = 1 ounce
- 1 kg = 2.2 lb

Household to household (also known as standard)

Volume

- 60 drops = 1 tsp
- 3 tsp = 1 tbsp
- 6 tsp = 1 oz
- 2 tbsp = 1 oz
- 8 oz = 1 c
- 2 c = 1 pt
- 4 c = 1 qt

Metric to metric

Volume

- 0.001 L = 1 milliliter
- 0.01 L = 1 centiliter
- 0.1 L = 1 deciliter
- 1 L = 1,000 mL
- 10 L = 1 dekaliter
- 100 L = 1 hectoliter
- 1,000 L = 1 kiloliter

Weight

- 0.001 g = 1 mg
- 0.01 g = 1 centigram
- 0.1 g = 1 decigram

- 1 g = 1,000 mg
- 10 g = 1 dekagram
- 100 g = 1 hectogram
- 1,000 g = 1 kilogram

Converting Within the Metric System

When you convert a quantity from one unit of metric measurement to another, you should

1. Move the decimal point to the right when you convert from a larger to a smaller unit. This is dividing.
2. Move the decimal point to the left when you convert from a smaller to a larger unit. This is multiplying.

Drawing a Drug from an Ampule

CRITICAL PROCEDURE STEPS

1. Identify your patient, wash your hands, and put on gloves.
2. Gently tap the top of the ampule to settle the liquid to the bottom of the ampule.
3. Wipe the ampule's neck with an alcohol swab.
4. Wrap a 2 × 2 gauze pad around the ampule's neck and snap the neck away from you.
5. Insert the filtered needle into the ampule without touching the side of the ampule.
6. Pull back on the plunger to aspirate the liquid completely into the syringe.
7. Replace with the regular needle and push the plunger until the medication just reaches the tip of the needle.

Drug Calculation Formulas

Basic formula

$$\text{amount to administer} = \frac{\text{desired dose}}{\text{dose on hand}} \times \text{quantity of dose on hand}$$

By weight

Ordered: Erythromycin 40 mg/kg/day po q4h. Patient weighs 34 lb.

1. Convert the patient's weight to kilograms using the proportion method. For accuracy when converting, round to the nearest hundredth (two decimal places).

   a. Set up the proportion. (Recall 1 kg = 2.2 lb.)

   $$\frac{34 \text{ lb}}{x} = \frac{2.2 \text{ lb}}{1 \text{ kg}}$$

   b. Cross multiply. Remember to multiply the bottom left number by the top right number and multiply the top left number by the bottom right number:

   $$x \times 2.2 \text{ lb} = 34 \text{ lb} \times 1 \text{ kg}$$

   c. Solve for x.

   $$x = \frac{34}{2.2}$$

   $$x = 15.45 \text{ kg}$$

2. Calculate the desired dose (D) for 24 hours by multiplying the dose ordered by the weight in kilograms.

   $$40 \text{ mg} \times 15.45 \text{ kg} = \text{desired dose } (D) \text{ for 24 hours}$$
   $$618 \text{ mg} = D \text{ (amount of medication to give in 24 hours)}$$

3. Calculate the desired dose (*D*) for one dose by dividing the amount to be received by the number of times the medication will be received in 24 hours.

   In this case, the medication is to be given six times in 24 hours.

$$618 \text{ mg divided by } 6 = 103 \text{ mg}$$
(desired dose for one dose)

4. Calculate the amount of medication to administer using the formula or the proportion method.

Proportion method

1. Set up the first fraction with the amount of drug ordered over the unknown (in this case, the number of capsules):

$$\frac{30 \text{ mg}}{x}$$

2. Set up the second fraction with the amount of drug in a single capsule and a single capsule (dosage unit):

$$\frac{10 \text{ mg}}{1 \text{ cap}}$$

3. Then use both fractions in a proportion, making sure the same units of measure are on the top and bottom of each side of the proportion.

$$\frac{30 \text{ mg}}{x} = \frac{10 \text{ mg}}{1 \text{ cap}}$$

4. Cross multiply. Multiply the bottom left number by the top right number, and multiply the top left number by the bottom right number:

$$x \times 10 \text{ mg} = 30 \text{ mg} \times 1 \text{ cap}$$

5. To solve for x, divide both sides of the equation by 10 mg; then do the arithmetic, canceling out like terms in the top and bottom of each fraction:

$$\frac{x \times \cancel{10\text{ mg}}}{\cancel{10\text{ mg}}} = \frac{30\text{ mg} \times 1\text{ cap}}{10\text{ mg}}$$

$$x = \frac{30\text{ caps}}{10}$$

$$x = 3\text{ caps}$$

Drug Categories and Actions for Commonly Prescribed Drugs

Drug Category	Action of Drug	Generic Name (Trade Name) Examples*
Analgesic	Relieves mild to severe pain	Acetaminophen (Tylenol®); acetylsalicylic acid, or aspirin; morphine sulfate (MS Contin®)*; oxycodone HCl (Oxycontin®)*
Anesthetic	Prevents sensation of pain (generally, locally, or topically)	Lidocaine HCl (Xylocaine®, Lidoderm®)*; tetracaine HCl (Pontocaine®)
Antacid/antiulcer	Neutralizes stomach acid	Calcium carbonate (Tums®); esomeprazole (Nexium®); lansoprazole (Prevacid®); pantoprazole sodium (Protonix®)*
Anthelmintic	Kills, paralyzes, or inhibits the growth of parasitic worms	Mebendazole (Vermox®); pyrantel pamoate (Combantrin®, Antiminth®)
Antidysrhythmic (antiarrhythmic)	Normalizes heartbeat in cases of certain cardiac dysrhythmias	Disopyramide phosphate (Norpace®); propafenone HCl (Rythmol®); propranolol HCl (Inderal®)

continued

*Indicates top 200 commonly prescribed drug in the year 2014.

103

Drug Category	Action of Drug	Generic Name (Trade Name) Examples*
Antiasthmatic	Treats or prevents asthma attacks	Montelukast (Singulair®)*; fluticasone propionate/salmeterol (Advair Diskus®)*; albuterol (ProAir HFA®)*
Antibiotic (antibacterial)	Kills bacterial microorganisms or inhibits their growth	Amoxicillin (Amoxil®)*; azithromycin (Zithromax®)*; cefprozil (Cefzil®); ciprofloxacin (Cipro®)*; clarithromycin (Biaxin XL®); clindamycin (Cleocin®)*
Anticholinergic	Blocks parasympathetic nerve impulses	Atropine sulfate (Isopto Atropine®); dicyclomine HCl (Bentyl®); ipratropium (Atrovent®)
Anticoagulant	Prevents blood from clotting	Enoxaparin sodium (Lovenox®); heparin sodium (Hep-Lock®); warfarin sodium (Coumadin®)*
Anticonvulsant	Relieves or controls seizures (convulsions)	Clonazepam (Klonopin®)*; divalproex sodium (Depakote®); phenobarbital sodium (Luminal® Sodium); phenytoin (Dilantin®)

Antidepressant (four types)	Relieves depression	
Tricyclic		Amitriptyline HCl (Elavil®); doxepin HCl (Sinequan®)
Monoamine oxidase inhibitor (MAOI)		Phenelzine sulfate (Nardil®); tranylcypromine sulfate (Parnate®)
Selective serotonin reuptake inhibitor (SSRI)		Escitalopram (Lexapro®)*; fluoxetine HCl (Prozac®); paroxetine HCl (Paxil®)*; sertraline HCl (Zoloft®)*
Serotonin-norepinephrine reuptake inhibitor (SNRI)		Venlafaxine HCl (Effexor XR®)*; duloxetine HCl (Cymbalta®)*
Antidiabetic	Treats diabetes by reducing glucose	Metformin (Glucophage®)*; glipizide (Glucotrol®)*; pioglitazone HCl (Actos®)*; insulin glargine (Lantus®)*

continued

Drug Category	Action of Drug	Generic Name (Trade Name) Examples*
Antidiarrheal	Relieves diarrhea	Bismuth subsalicylate (Pepto-Bismol®); kaolin and pectin mixtures (Kaopectate®); loperamide HCl (Imodium®)
Antiemetic	Prevents or relieves nausea and vomiting	Prochlorperazine (Compazine®); promethazine (Phenergan®); trimethobenzamide HCl (Tigan®)
Antifungal	Kills or inhibits growth of fungi	Amphotericin B (Fungizone®); fluconazole (Diflucan®)*; nystatin (Mycostatin®); terbinafine (Lamisil®)
Antihistamine	Counteracts effects of histamine and relieves allergy symptoms	Cetirizine HCl (Zyrtec®)*; diphenhydramine HCl (Benadryl®); fexofenadine (Allegra®); desloratadine (Clarinex®)
Antihypertensive	Reduces blood pressure	Amlodipine (Norvasc®)*; diltiazem HCl (Cartia XL®); quinapril lisinopril (Accupril) (Prinivil)*; metoprolol succinate (Toprol XL®)*; valsartan (Diovan®)*

Anti-inflammatory (two types)	Reduces inflammation	
Nonsteroidal (NSAID)		Naproxen (Aleve®)*; colchicine (Colcrys®)**; ibuprofen (Motrin®, Advil®)*; celecoxib (Celebrex®)*
Steroid		Dexamethasone (Decadron®); methylprednisolone (Medrol®)*; prednisone (Deltasone™)*; triamcinolone (Kenalog®)*
Antilipemic (antilipidemic)	Lowers blood lipids such as triglycerides	Gemfibrozil (Lopid®); atorvastatin (Lipitor®)*; fenofibrate (TriCor®)*; ezetimibe/simvastatin (Vytorin®)*; ezetimibe (Zetia®)*; rosuvastatin (Crestor®)*
Antineoplastic	Poisons cancerous cells	Bleomycin sulfate (Blenoxane®); dactinomycin (Cosmegen®); paclitaxel (Taxol®); tamoxifen citrate (Nolvadex®)

continued

Drug Category	Action of Drug	Generic Name (Trade Name) Examples*
Antipsychotic	Controls psychotic symptoms	Chlorpromazine HCl (Thorazine®), clozapine (Clozaril®); haloperidol (Haldol®); risperidone (Risperdal®)*; thioridazine HCl (Mellaril®)
Antipyretic	Reduces fever	Acetaminophen (Tylenol®); acetylsalicylic acid, or aspirin
Antiseptic	Inhibits growth of microorganisms	Isopropyl alcohol; 70% povidone-iodine (Betadine®); chlorhexidine gluconate (PerioChip®)®
Antitussive	Inhibits cough reflex	Codeine; dextromethorphan hydrobromide (component of Robitussin® DM)
Bronchodilator	Dilates bronchi (airways in the lungs)	Albuterol (Proventil®)*; epinephrine (Epinephrine Mist®); salmeterol (Serevent®); tiotropium bromide (Spiriva®)*
Cathartic (laxative)	Induces defecation, alleviates constipation	Bisacodyl (Dulcolax®); casanthranol (Peri-Colace®); magnesium hydroxide (Milk of Magnesia®)
Contraceptive	Reduces risk of pregnancy	Ethinyl estradiol and norgestimate (Ortho Tri-Cyclen®); norethindrone and ethinyl estradiol (Loestrin® 24 Fe)*; norgestrel (Ovrette®)

Decongestant	Relieves nasal swelling and congestion	Oxymetazoline HCl (Afrin®); phenylephrine HCl (Neo-Synephrine®); pseudoephedrine HCl (Sudafed®)
Diuretic	Increases urine output, reduces blood pressure and cardiac output	Bumetanide (Bumex®); furosemide (Lasix®)*; hydrochlorothiazide (HydroDIURIL®)*; mannitol (Osmitrol®); spironolactone (Aldactone®)
Expectorant	Liquefies mucus in bronchi; allows expectoration of sputum, mucus, and phlegm	Guaifenesin (Mucinex®)
Hemostatic	Controls or stops bleeding by promoting coagulation	Aminocaproic acid (Amicar®); phytonadione or vitamin K₁ (Mephyton®); thrombin (Thrombogen®)
Hormone replacement	Replaces or resolves hormone deficiency	Insulin (Humulin®) for pancreatic deficiency; levothyroxine sodium (Synthroid®)* for thyroid deficiency; conjugated estrogens (Premarin Tabs®)*

continued

Drug Category	Action of Drug	Generic Name (Trade Name) Examples*
Hypnotic (sleep-inducing) or sedative	Induces sleep or relaxation (depending on drug potency and dosage)	Chloral hydrate (Noctec®); secobarbital sodium (Seconal Sodium®); zolpidem (Ambien®)*
Muscle relaxant	Relaxes skeletal muscles	Carisoprodol (Rela® or Soma®); cyclobenzaprine HCl (Flexeril®)*
Mydriatic	Constricts vessels of eye or nasal passage, raises blood pressure, dilates pupil of eye in ophthalmic preparations	Atropine sulfate (Atropisol) for ophthalmic use; phenylephrine HCl (Alcon Efrin) for ophthalmic use or (Neo-Synephrine®) for nasal use
Stimulant (central nervous system)	Increases activity of brain and other organs, decreases appetite	Amphetamine sulfate (Benzedrine Amphetamine sulfate); caffeine (No-Doz®); also a component of many analgesic formulations and coffee
Vasoconstrictor	Constricts blood vessels, increases blood pressure	Dopamine HCl (Intropin®); norepinephrine bitartrate (Levophed®)
Vasodilator	Dilates blood vessels, decreases blood pressure	Enalopril (Vasotec®); lisinopril (Prinivil®)*; nitroglycerin (Nitrostat®, NitroQuick®)

Source: RxList (http://www.rxlist.com).

Inhalation Therapy

CRITICAL PROCEDURE STEPS

1. Identify the patient and wash your hands.
2. Check the medication rights.
3. Check the package insert and prepare the medication as directed.
4. Shake the container as directed and share this information with the patient.

Nasal Inhaler

Instruct the patient as follows:

5. Blow your nose.
6. Tilt your head back slightly and insert the tip of the inhaler into the nose ½ inch.
7. Point the tip straight up toward the inner corner of the eye.
8. Use the opposite hand to block the other nostril.
9. Inhale gently while quickly and firmly squeezing the inhaler.
10. Remove the inhaler tip and breathe through the mouth.
11. Shake the inhaler and repeat the process for the other nostril.
12. Keep your head tilted back and do not blow your nose for several minutes (if indicated in the package insert).

Oral Inhaler

Instruct the patient as follows:

5. Warm the canister by rolling it in the palms of your hands.

continued

6. Assemble the inhaler as directed in the package insert.

7. Hold your mouth open and place the inhaler as instructed in the package insert.

8. Exhale normally and inhale through the canister as you depress it.

9. You must be inhaling when the canister is depressed.

10. Breathe in until your lungs are full and hold your breath for 10 seconds.

11. Breathe out normally.

12. Repeat the process if additional "puffs" are prescribed.

After Giving an Inhalation Medication

13. Remain with the patient to monitor for changes and possible adverse reactions.

14. Recap and secure the medication container.

15. Instruct the patient in this procedure.

16. Wash your hands.

17. Give the patient an information sheet about the drug.

18. Discuss the information with the patient and answer any questions.

19. Document the date, time, drug name, dosage, expiration date, lot number, manufacturer, route, site, significant patient reactions, and patient education in the chart.

Types of Injections

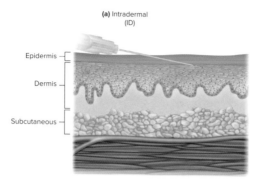

(a) Intradermal (ID)

Epidermis

Dermis

Subcutaneous

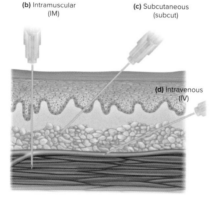

(b) Intramuscular (IM)

(c) Subcutaneous (subcut)

(d) Intravenous (IV)

Intradermal (ID)

- Administer in the upper layers of the skin.
- Common sites are the forearm and the back.
- Avoid scarred, blemished, or hairy areas.

Intramuscular (IM)

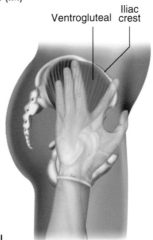

Ventrogluteal

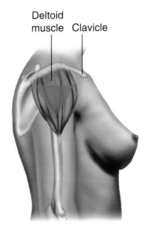

Deltoid

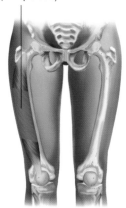

Vastus lateralis
(mid-portion)

Vastus lateralis

Subcutaneous (subcut)

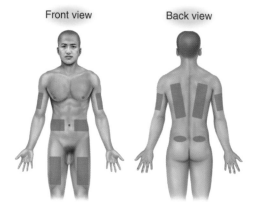

Front view

Back view

Injection Techniques

Intradermal (ID)

CRITICAL PROCEDURE STEPS

1. Identify the patient.
2. Wash your hands and put on gloves.
3. Check the medication rights against the physician's order.
4. Identify the injection site, usually the forearm.
5. Prepare the skin with an alcohol swab, moving in a circle from the center out.
6. Let the skin dry before giving the injection.
7. Hold the patient's forearm and stretch the skin tight with one hand.
8. Place the needle, bevel up, almost flat against the skin and insert the needle.
9. Inject the drug gently and slowly until a wheal is raised.
10. After the full dose of the drug has been injected, withdraw the needle.
11. Properly dispose of the used materials and the needle and syringe immediately.
12. Remove the gloves and wash your hands.
13. Stay with the patient to monitor for unexpected reactions.
14. Document the injection with the date, time, drug name, dosage, expiration date, lot number, manufacturer, route, site, significant patient reactions, and any patient education in the patient's chart.

CRITICAL PROCEDURE STEPS

1. Identify the patient.
2. Wash your hands and put on gloves.
3. Check the medication rights.
4. Prepare the drug and draw up the amount ordered.
5. Choose a site and gently tap it.
6. Clean the site with an alcohol swab, moving in a circle from the center out.
7. Let the skin dry before giving the injection.
8. Stretch the skin taut over the injection site.
9. Insert the needle with a quick, dart-like thrust at a 90-degree angle.
10. Release the skin and aspirate to check needle placement.
11. Slowly inject the drug if the needle is placed correctly (no blood appears when you aspirate).
12. After injecting the full dose of the drug, place a 2 × 2 piece of gauze over the injection site.
13. Quickly remove the needle at a 90-degree angle.
14. Use the 2 × 2 piece of gauze to apply pressure to the site and massage it, if indicated.
15. Properly dispose of used materials and the needle and syringe.
16. Remove the gloves and wash your hands.
17. Stay with the patient to monitor for unexpected reactions.
18. Document the injection with the date, time, drug name, dosage, expiration date, lot number, manufacturer, route, site, significant patient reactions, and any patient education in the patient's chart.

CRITICAL PROCEDURE STEPS

1. Identify the patient.
2. Wash your hands and put on gloves.
3. Check the medication rights.
4. Prepare the drug and draw up the amount ordered.
5. Choose a site.
6. Clean the site with an alcohol swab, moving in a circle from the center out.
7. Let the skin dry before giving the injection.
8. Pinch the skin firmly to lift the subcutaneous tissue.
9. Position the needle, bevel up, at a 45-degree angle to the skin.
10. Insert the needle with one quick motion and release the skin.
11. Inject the drug slowly.
12. After injecting the full dose of the drug, place a 2 × 2 piece of gauze over the injection site and withdraw the needle.
13. Apply pressure at the puncture site with the gauze.
14. Massage the site gently, if indicated.
15. Properly dispose of used materials and the needle and syringe.
16. Remove the gloves and wash your hands.
17. Stay with the patient to monitor for unexpected reactions.

18. Document the injection with the date, time, drug name, dosage, expiration date, lot number, manufacturer, route, site, significant patient reactions, and any patient education in the patient's chart.

Pediatric Patients

Giving injections

- Distract the child by talking to him or her.
- Praise the child.
- Use a topical anesthetic.
- Avoid letting the child see the syringe.
- Be swift.

Oral medication guidelines

YOU SHOULD KNOW

- Use a pediatric calibrated dropper to measure the amount ordered.
- Administer the medication to the side of the tongue.
- Hold the child until you are sure the medication has been swallowed.
- If a small amount dribbles out, do not give additional medication.
- If the child vomits within 5 minutes and you can see the medication in the vomit, administer more medication. If you are unsure, consult the physician.
- If the medication comes only in tablet form, check a drug reference to see if it can be crushed and given with food.

Pregnancy and Lactation Drug Label Requirements (June 2015)

The FDA requires the following information on prescription drug labels to assist the prescriber and the patient in determining the risks and benefits of each.

Category	Label Requirements
Pregnancy (includes Labor and Delivery)	– Pregnancy/fetal risk summary – Clinical considerations and data – Inadvertent exposure considerations – Prescribing decisions for pregnant patients – Information for the pregnancy exposure registry when available
Lacation (includes Nursing Mothers)	– Information about the amount of drug in the breast milk – Information about potential effects of the drug on the breastfed infant
Females and Males of Reproductive Potential	– Need for pregacy testing when taking the drug – Contraception recommendations – Information about infertility as it relates to the drug

Reconstituting and Drawing a Drug

CRITICAL PROCEDURE STEPS

1. Wash your hands and put on gloves.
2. Place the drug vial and the diluent on the countertop. Wipe each with an alcohol swab.

3. Using a syringe and needle, pull the plunger back on the syringe to the amount of diluent needed to reconstitute the drug ordered.
4. Puncture the diluent vial and inject the air into the diluent.
5. Invert the vial and aspirate the diluent.
6. Remove the needle from the diluent, inject the diluent into the drug vial, and withdraw the needle.
7. Properly dispose of the needle and syringe.
8. Roll the vial between your hands to mix it thoroughly.
9. Do not shake the vial unless directed to do so on the product label.
10. Prepare the second syringe and needle.
11. Pull back the plunger to the mark that reflects the amount of drug ordered.
12. Inject the air into the drug vial.
13. Invert the vial and aspirate the proper amount of drug into the syringe.

Rules for Drug Administration

YOU SHOULD KNOW

- Give only the medication the physician prescribes.
- Wash your hands before you handle the medication.
- Perform a triple check.
- Calculate the dose if necessary.

continued

- Avoid leaving a prepared drug unattended.
- Never administer a drug that someone else has prepared.
- Ensure correct patient identification.
- Ask the patient about drug allergies.
- Be sure the physician is in the office when you administer a drug or vaccine.
- Have the patient remain in the facility for 10 to 20 minutes after administering the drug.
- Give the patient information about the drug and its side effects.
- If the patient refuses to take the drug, discard it according to office policy.
- Do not flush the drug down the toilet or return it to its original container.
- Document the refusal and alert the physician.
- If you make an error in drug administration, tell the physician immediately.
- Document the drug and dose administered.
- Never document administration before giving the medication.

Z-Track Injections

Used for medications that might irritate the skin.

- Pull the skin to one side.
- Insert the needle.
- Inject the medication.
- Release the skin to close off the injection site.
- Do not massage the site.

Minor Surgery

Assisting as a Floater

CRITICAL PROCEDURE STEPS

1. Perform routine handwashing and put on exam gloves.

2. Monitor the patient during the procedure; record the results in the patient's chart.

3. During the surgery, assist as needed.

4. Add sterile items to the tray as necessary.

5. Pour sterile solution into a sterile bowl as needed.

6. Assist in administering additional anesthetic.

   a. Check the medication vial two times.

   b. Clean the rubber stopper with an alcohol pad (write the date opened when using a new bottle); leave pad on top.

   c. Present the needle and syringe to the doctor.

   d. Remove the alcohol pad from the vial, and show the label to the doctor.

   e. Hold the vial upside down and grasp the lower edge firmly; brace your wrist with your free hand.

   f. Allow the doctor to fill the syringe.

   g. Check the medication vial a final time.

7. Receive specimens for laboratory examination.

   a. Uncap the specimen container; present it to the doctor for the introduction of the specimen.

   b. Replace the cap and label the container.

   c. Treat all specimens as infectious.

continued

d. Place the specimen container in a transport bag or other container.

e. Complete the requisition form to send the specimen to the laboratory.

Assisting as a Sterile Scrub Assistant

CRITICAL PROCEDURE STEPS

1. Perform a surgical scrub and put on sterile gloves.
2. Remember to remove the sterile towel covering the sterile field and instruments before gloving.
3. Close and arrange the surgical instruments on the tray.
4. Prepare for swabbing by inserting gauze squares into the sterile dressing forceps.
5. Pass the instruments as necessary.
6. Swab the wound as requested.
7. Retract the wound as requested.
8. Cut the sutures as requested.

Assisting After Minor Surgery

CRITICAL PROCEDURE STEPS

1. Monitor the patient.
2. Put on clean exam gloves and clean the wound with antiseptic.

3. Dress the wound.
4. Remove the gloves and wash your hands.
5. Give the patient oral postoperative instructions in addition to the release packet.
6. Discharge the patient.
7. Put on clean exam gloves.
8. Properly dispose of used materials and disposable instruments.
9. Sanitize reusable instruments and prepare them for disinfection and/or sterilization as needed.
10. Clean equipment and the exam room according to OSHA guidelines.
11. Remove the gloves and wash your hands.

Basic Instruments

Cutting and dissecting

- **Curettes**—used for scraping tissue, come in a variety of shapes and sizes, and consist of a circular blade (loop) attached to a rod-shaped handle
- **Scalpels**—consist of a handle that holds a disposable blade; specific use determines the shape and size of the blade
- **Scissors**—may be straight or curved and have either blunt or pointed tips

Grasping and clamping instruments

- **Forceps**—used to grasp or hold objects; include thumb, tissue, and sponge forceps
- **Hemostats**—used to close off blood vessels; the handles lock on ratchets, holding the jaws securely closed

- **Towel clamps**—keep towels in place during a surgical procedure to help maintain a sterile field

Retracting, dilating, and probing instruments

- **Dilators**—slender, pointed instruments; used to enlarge a body opening, such as a tear duct
- **Probes**—a slender rod with a blunt tip shaped like a bulb; used to explore wounds or body cavities and to locate or clear blockages
- **Retractors**—allow greater access to and a better view of a surgical site; may be held open by hand or have ratchets or locks to keep them open

Suturing instruments

- **Needle holders**—special instrument to hold, insert, and retrieve suture needles
- **Suture needles**—carry suture material through the tissue being sutured; may be pointed or blunt at one end; straight or curved

Creating a Sterile Field

CRITICAL PROCEDURE STEPS

1. Clean and disinfect the tray or Mayo stand.
2. Wash your hands and assemble the necessary materials.
3. Check the label on the instrument pack to make sure it is the correct pack for the procedure.
4. Check the date and sterilization indicator on the instrument pack to make sure the pack is still sterile.

5. Place the sterile pack on the tray or stand, and unfold the outermost fold away from yourself.

6. Unfold the sides of the pack outward, touching only the areas that will become the underside of the sterile field.

7. Open the final flap toward yourself, stepping back and away from the sterile field.

8. Place additional packaged sterile items on the sterile field.

   a. Ensure that you have the correct item or instrument and that the package is still sterile.

   b. Stand away from the sterile field.

   c. Grasp the package flaps and pull apart about halfway.

   d. Bring the corners of the wrapping beneath the package, paying attention not to contaminate the inner package or item.

   e. Hold the package over the sterile field with the opening down; with a quick movement, pull the flap completely open and snap the sterile item onto the field.

9. Place basins and bowls near the edge of the sterile field so that you can pour liquids without reaching over the field.

10. Use sterile transfer forceps if necessary to add additional items to the sterile field.

11. If necessary, don sterile gloves after a sterile scrub to arrange items on the sterile field.

Performing a Surgical Scrub

CRITICAL PROCEDURE STEPS

1. Remove all jewelry and roll up your sleeves to above the elbow.
2. Assemble the necessary materials.
3. Turn on the faucet using the foot or knee pedal.
4. Wet your hands from the fingertips to the elbows. You must keep your hands higher than your elbows.
5. Under running water, use a sterile brush to clean under your fingernails.
6. Apply surgical soap and scrub your hands, fingers, areas between the fingers, wrists, and forearms with the scrub sponge, using a firm, circular motion. Follow the manufacturer's recommendations to determine appropriate length of time, usually 2–6 minutes.
7. Rinse from fingers to elbows, always keeping your hands higher than your elbows.
8. Thoroughly dry your hands and forearms with sterile towels, working from the hands to the elbows.
9. Turn off the faucet with the foot or knee pedal. Use a sterile towel if a foot or knee pedal is not used.

Donning Sterile Gloves

CRITICAL PROCEDURE STEPS

1. Obtain the correct size gloves.
2. Check the package for tears and ensure that the expiration date has not passed.

3. Perform a surgical scrub.
4. Peel the outer wrap from gloves and place the inner wrapper on a clean surface above waist level.
5. Position gloves so that the cuff end is closest to your body.
6. Touch only the flaps as you open the package.
7. Use instructions provided on the inner package, if available.
8. Do not reach over the sterile inside of the inner package.
9. Follow these steps if there are no instructions:
   a. Open the package so that the first flap is opened away from you.
   b. Pinch the corner and pull to one side.
   c. Put your fingertips under the side flaps and gently pull until the package is completely open.
10. Use your nondominant hand to grasp the inside cuff of the opposite glove without touching the outside of the glove.
11. Holding the glove at arm's length and waist level, insert the dominant hand into the glove with the palm facing up. Don't let the outside of the glove touch any other surface.
12. With your sterile gloved hand, slip the gloved fingers into the cuff of the other glove.
13. Pick up the other glove, touching only the outside. Don't touch any other surfaces.
14. Pull the glove up and onto your hand. Ensure that the sterile gloved hand does not touch skin.
15. Adjust your fingers as necessary, touching only glove to glove.

continued

16. Do not adjust the cuffs because your forearms may contaminate the gloves.

17. Keep your hands in front of you, between your shoulders and waist. If you move your hands out of this area, they are considered contaminated.

18. If contamination or the possibility of contamination occurs, change gloves.

19. Remove gloves the same way you remove clean gloves, by touching only the inside.

Rules for Keeping a Field Sterile

YOU SHOULD KNOW

A sterile field is considered contaminated and must be redone if

- An unsterile item touches the field.
- Someone reaches across the field.
- The field becomes wet.
- The field is left unattended and uncovered.
- You turn your back on the field.

Rules for Sterile Technique

YOU SHOULD KNOW

1. Do not touch a nonsterile article to a sterile article or area. This will cause the sterile area or article to be considered nonsterile.

2. If you are unsure about the sterility of an article or area, consider it nonsterile.

3. Unused, opened sterile supplies must be discarded or resterilized.

4. Packages must be wrapped or sealed in such a way that they can be opened without contamination.

5. The edges of wrappers (1-inch margin) covering sterile supplies and the outer lips of bottles and flasks containing sterile solutions are not considered sterile.

6. If a sterile surface or package becomes wet, it is considered contaminated and should not be used.

7. Do not reach over a sterile field when you are not wearing sterile clothing. This action contaminates the sterile field.

8. Keep your hands between your shoulders and your waist when wearing sterile gloves to maintain sterility.

9. Do not turn your back on a sterile field even if you are in a sterile gown. Your back is always considered contaminated.

Suture Removal

CRITICAL PROCEDURE STEPS

1. Clean and disinfect the tray or Mayo stand.

2. Wash your hands and assemble the necessary materials.

3. Check the date and sterilization indicator on the suture removal pack.

4. Unwrap the suture removal pack and place it on the tray or stand to create a sterile field.

continued

5. Unwrap the sterile bowls and add them to the sterile field.

6. Pour a small amount of antiseptic solution into one bowl, and pour a small amount of hydrogen peroxide into the other bowl.

7. Cover the tray with a sterile towel to protect the sterile field while you are out of the room.

8. Escort the patient to the exam room and explain the procedure.

9. Perform a routine handwash, remove the towel from the tray, and put on exam gloves.

10. Remove the old dressing.
    a. Lift the tape toward the middle of the dressing to avoid pulling on the wound.
    b. If the dressing adheres to the wound, cover the dressing with gauze squares soaked in hydrogen peroxide. Leave the wet gauze in place for several seconds to loosen the dressing.
    c. Save the old dressing for the doctor to inspect.

11. Inspect the wound for signs of infection.

12. Clean the wound with gauze pads soaked in antiseptic, and pat it dry with clean gauze pads.

13. Remove the gloves and wash your hands.

14. Notify the doctor that the wound is ready for examination.

15. Once the doctor indicates that the wound is sufficiently healed to proceed, put on clean exam gloves.

16. Place a square of gauze next to the wound for collecting the sutures as they are removed.

17. Sutures: Grasp the first suture knot with forceps. Staples: Slide the staple remover under the first staple.

18. Sutures: Gently lift the knot away from the skin to allow room for the suture scissors. Staples: Gently press down on the staple remover handle.

19. Sutures: Slide the suture scissors under the suture material, and cut the suture where it enters the skin. Staples: Continue pressing down on the staple remover to straighten the staple so that it exits the skin.

20. Sutures: Gently lift the knot up and toward the wound to remove the suture without opening the wound. Staples: Observe the staple on each side to ensure that it is completely out of the skin.

21. Place the suture or staple on the gauze pad and inspect to ensure that the entire suture or staple is present.

22. Repeat the removal process until all sutures or staples have been removed.

23. Count the sutures or staples and compare the number with the number indicated in the patient's record.

24. Clean the wound with antiseptic and allow the wound to air-dry.

25. Dress the wound as ordered, or notify the doctor if sterile strips or butterfly closures are to be applied.

26. Observe the patient for signs of distress, such as wincing or grimacing.

27. Properly dispose of used materials and disposable instruments.

28. Remove the gloves and wash your hands.

continued

29. Instruct the patient on wound care.

30. In the patient's chart, record pertinent information, such as the condition of the wound and the type of closures used, if any.

31. Escort the patient to the checkout area.

32. Put on clean gloves.

33. Sanitize reusable instruments and prepare them for disinfection and/or sterilization as needed.

34. Clean the equipment and exam room according to OSHA guidelines.

35. Remove the gloves and wash your hands.

Wounds

Care—promoting healing

- Clean debris from nonsurgical wounds.
- Keep the wound dry.
- Sutured wounds heal more quickly.
- Clean a wound daily with a mild antiseptic or soap and water.

Indications for physician's care

Patients with any of the following should seek the care of a physician:

- Jagged or gaping edges
- A face wound
- Limited movement in the area of the wound
- Tenderness or inflammation at the wound site
- Purulent drainage

- A fever greater than 100°F
- Red streaks near the wound
- A puncture wound
- Bleeding that does not stop after 10 minutes of pressure
- Sutures or staples coming out on their own or too early

Wrapping Surgical Instruments

CRITICAL PROCEDURE STEPS

1. Wash your hands and put on gloves before beginning to wrap the items to be sterilized.

2. Place a square of paper or muslin on the table with one point toward you. With muslin, use a double thickness. The paper or fabric must be large enough to allow all four points to cover the instruments or equipment you will be wrapping. It must also be large enough to provide an overlap, which will be used as a handling flap.

3. Place each item to be included in the pack in the center area of the paper or fabric "diamond." Items that will be used together should be wrapped together. Take care, however, that surfaces of the items do not touch each other inside the pack. Inspect each item to make sure it is operating correctly. Place hinged instruments in the pack in the open position. Wrap a small piece of paper, muslin, or gauze around delicate edges or points to protect against damage to other instruments or to the pack wrapping.

4. Place a sterilization indicator inside the pack with the instruments. Position the indicator correctly, following the manufacturer's guidelines.

continued

135

5. Fold the bottom point of the diamond up and over the instruments in to the center. Fold back a small portion of the point.

6. Fold the right point of the diamond in to the center. Again, fold back a small portion of the point to be used as a handle.

7. Fold the left point of the diamond in to the center, folding back a small portion to form a handle. The pack should now resemble an open envelope.

8. Grasp the covered instruments (the bottom of the envelope) and fold this portion up, toward the top point. Fold the top point down over the pack, making sure the pack is snug but not too tight.

9. Secure the pack with autoclave tape. A "quick-opening tab" can be created by folding a small portion of the tape back onto itself. The pack must be snug enough to prevent instruments from slipping out of the wrapping or damaging each other inside the pack but loose enough to allow adequate circulation of steam through the pack.

10. Label the pack with your initials and the date. List the contents of the pack as well. If the pack contains syringes, be sure to identify the syringe size(s).

11. Place the pack aside for loading into the autoclave.

12. Remove gloves, dispose of them in the appropriate waste container, and wash your hands.

For wrapping instruments and equipment in bags or envelopes:

1. Wash your hands and put on gloves before beginning to wrap the items to be sterilized.

2. Insert the items into the bag or envelope as indicated by the manufacturer's directions. Hinged instruments should be opened before insertion into the package.

3. Close and seal the pack. Make sure the sterilization indicator is not damaged or already exposed.

4. Label the pack with your initials and the date. List the contents of the pack as well. The pens or pencils used to label the pack must be waterproof; otherwise, the contents of the pack and date of sterilization will be obliterated.

5. Place the pack aside for loading into the autoclave.

6. Remove gloves, dispose of them in the appropriate waste container, and wash your hands.

Nutrition

Alerting Patients with Food Allergies to the Dangers of Common Foods

CRITICAL PROCEDURE STEPS

1. Identify the patient and introduce yourself.

2. Discuss the results of the patient's allergy tests (if available), reinforcing the licensed practitioner's instructions. Provide the patient with a checklist of the foods the patient has been found to be allergic to and review the list with the patient.

continued

3. Discuss with the patient the possible allergic reactions those foods can cause.

4. Talk about how the patient can avoid or eliminate those foods from the diet. Point out that the patient needs to be alert to avoid the allergy-causing foods not only in their basic forms but also as ingredients in prepared dishes and packaged foods. (Patients allergic to peanuts, for example, should avoid products containing peanut oil as well as peanuts.)

5. Tell the patient to read labels carefully and to inquire at restaurants about the use of those ingredients in dishes listed on the menu.

6. With the licensed practitioner's or dietitian's consent, talk with the patient about the possibility of finding adequate substitutes for the foods if they are among the patient's favorites. Also discuss, if necessary, how the patient can obtain the nutrients in those foods from other sources (for example, the need for extra calcium sources if the patient is allergic to dairy products). Provide these explanations to the patient in writing, if appropriate, along with supplementary materials such as recipe pamphlets, a list of resources for obtaining food substitutes, and so on.

7. Discuss with the patient the procedures to follow if the allergy-causing foods are accidentally ingested.

8. Answer the patient's questions and remind the patient that you and the rest of the medical team are available if any questions or problems arise later on.

9. Document the patient education session or interchange in the patient's chart, indicate the patient's understanding, and initial the entry.

Calories Burned per Hour in Selected Activities

Moderate Physical Activity	Approximate Calories/Hr for a 154-lb Person*
Hiking	370
Light gardening/yard work	330
Dancing	330
Golf (walking and carrying clubs)	330
Bicycling (<10 mph)	290
Walking (3.5 mph)	280
Weight lifting (general light workout)	220
Stretching	180
Vigorous Physical Activity	Approximate Calories/Hr for a 154-lb Person*
Running/jogging (5 mph)	590
Bicycling (>10 mph)	590
Swimming (slow freestyle laps)	510
Aerobics	480
Walking (4.5 mph)	460
Heavy yard work (chopping wood)	440

continued

Vigorous Physical Activity	Approximate Calories/Hr for a 154-lb Person*
Weight lifting (vigorous effort)	440
Basketball (vigorous)	440

*Calories burned per hour will be higher for persons who weigh more than 154 lb (70 kg) and lower for persons who weigh less.

Source: Dietary Guidelines for Americans 2010, US Department of Health and Human Services, US Department of Agriculture, http://www.cnpp.usda.gov/dietaryguidelines.

Food Label Terms

- **Low calorie**—less than or equal to 40 calories per serving
- **Reduced calorie**—at least 25% fewer calories per serving than the food it replaces
- **Cholesterol free**—less than or equal to 2 mg cholesterol per serving
- **Low cholesterol**—less than or equal to 20 mg cholesterol per serving
- **Reduced cholesterol**—at least 25% less cholesterol per serving than the food it replaces
- **Low fat**—less than or equal to 3 g fat per serving
- **Reduced fat**—at least 25% less fat per serving than the food it replaces
- **Sodium free**—less than or equal to 5 mg sodium per serving
- **Very low sodium**—less than or equal to 35 mg sodium per serving
- **Low sodium**—less than or equal to 140 mg sodium per serving
- **Reduced sodium**—at least 25% less sodium per serving than the food it replaces

Saturated Fat and Cholesterol Sources

Food	Saturated Fat	Cholesterol
Cheddar cheese (1 oz)	6.0 g	30 mg
Mozzarella, part skim (1 oz)	3.1 g	15 mg
Whole milk (1 c)	5.1 g	33 mg
Skim milk (1 c)	0.3 g	4 mg
Butter (1 tbsp)	7.1 g	31 mg
Mayonnaise (1 tbsp)	1.7 g	8 mg
Tuna in oil (3 oz)	1.4 g	55 mg
Tuna in water (3 oz)	0.3 g	48 mg
Lean ground beef, broiled (3 oz)	6.2 g	74 mg
Leg of lamb, roasted (3 oz)	5.6 g	78 mg
Bacon (3 slices)	3.3 g	16 mg
Chicken breast, roasted (3 oz)	0.9 g	73 mg

Source: US Department of Agriculture.

Serving Sizes

Group	Quantity
Bread, cereal, rice, pasta	• 1 slice bread • 1 oz ready-to-eat cereal • ½ c cooked cereal, rice, or pasta
Vegetable	• 1 c raw leafy vegetables • ½ c other vegetables • ¾ c vegetable juice
Fruit	• 1 medium apple, banana, or orange • ½ c chopped, cooked, or canned fruit • ¾ c fruit juice
Milk, yogurt, cheese	• 1 c milk or yogurt • 1½ oz natural cheese • 2 oz processed cheese
Meat, poultry, fish, dry beans, eggs, and nuts	• 2–3 oz cooked lean meat, poultry, or fish • ½ c cooked dry beans or 1 egg counts as 1 oz lean meat • 2 tbsp peanut butter or ⅓ c nuts counts as 1 oz meat

Teaching a Patient to Read a Food Label

CRITICAL PROCEDURE STEPS

1. Identify the patient and introduce yourself.

2. Explain that food labels can be used as a valuable source of information when planning or implementing a prescribed diet.

3. Using a label from a food package, point out the Nutrition Facts section.

4. Describe the various elements on the label.

   - Serving size is the basis for the nutrition information provided.

   - Calories and calories from fat show the proportion of fat calories in the product.

   - The % Daily Value section shows how many grams (g) or milligrams (mg) of a variety of nutrients are contained in one serving. Then the label shows the percentage (%) of the recommended daily intake of each given nutrient (assuming a diet of 2,000 calories per day).

   - Recommendations for total amounts of various nutrients for both a 2,000-calorie and a 2,500-calorie diet are shown in chart form on the label. These numbers provide the basis for the daily value percentages.

   - Ingredients are listed in order from largest quantity to smallest quantity.

5. Inform the patient that a variety of similar products with significantly different nutritional values are often available. Explain that patients can use nutrition labels to evaluate and compare similar products. Patients must consider what a product contributes

continued

to their diets, not simply what it lacks. To do this, patients must read the entire label.

6. Ask the patient to compare two similar products and determine which would fit in better as part of a healthy, nutritious diet that meets that patient's individual needs.

7. Document the patient education session in the patient's chart, indicate the patient's understanding, and initial the entry.

USDA 2015 Dietary Guidelines Key Recommendations

Balancing calories to manage weight	• Promote healthy weight through improved eating and physical activity behaviors.
	• Control total calorie intake to manage body weight. For people who are overweight or obese, this will mean consuming fewer calories from foods and beverages.
	• Increase physical activity and reduce time spent in sedentary behaviors.
	• Maintain appropriate calorie balance during each stage of life: childhood, adolescence, adulthood, pregnancy and breast-feeding, and older age.
Foods and food components to reduce	• Reduce daily sodium intake to less than 2,300 milligrams (mg). Further reduce intake to 1,500 mg among people who are 51 and older and those of any age who are African American or have hypertension, diabetes, or chronic kidney disease.
	• Consume less than 10% of calories from saturated fatty acids by replacing them with monounsaturated and polyunsaturated fatty acids.
	• Consume less than 300 mg per day of dietary cholesterol.

continued

- Keep trans fatty acid consumption as low as possible by limiting foods that contain synthetic sources of trans fats and by limiting other solid fats.

- Reduce the intake of calories from solid fats and added sugars, but do not increase the use of low-calorie sweeteners to reduce sugar intake.

- Limit the consumption of foods that contain refined grains, especially refined grain foods that contain solid fats, added sugars, and sodium.

- If alcohol is consumed, it should be consumed in moderation (up to one drink per day for women and two drinks per day for men) and only by adults of legal drinking age.

Food and nutrients to increase (within calorie needs)	• Increase vegetable and fruit intake.
	• Eat a variety of vegetables, especially dark-green, red, and orange vegetables; beans; and peas.
	• Consume at least half of all grains as whole grains.
	• Increase intake of fat-free or low-fat milk and milk products.

	- Choose a variety of protein foods, which include seafood, lean meat and poultry, eggs, beans and peas, soy products, and unsalted nuts and seeds. - Increase the amount and variety of seafood consumed by choosing seafood in place of some meat and poultry. - Replace protein foods that are higher in solid fats with choices that are lower in solid fats and calories and/or are sources of oils. - Use oils to replace solid fats where possible. - Choose foods that provide more potassium, dietary fiber, calcium, and vitamin D, which are nutrients of concern in American diets.
Building healthy eating patterns	- Select an eating pattern that meets nutrient needs at an appropriate calorie level. - Monitor foods and beverages consumed, and assess their fit within a healthy eating pattern. - Follow food safety recommendations when preparing and eating foods.

Source: Adapted from "Dietary Guidelines for Americans 2015," US Department of Agriculture and US Department of Health and Human Services, http://www.dietaryguidelines.gov.

The USDA timeline says they will be out Fall 2015. LGW http://health.gov/dietaryguidelines/2015.asp#resources

Vitamins

Vitamin	Function
A	Aids in night vision; cell growth and maintenance; normal reproductive function; health of skin, mucous membranes, and intestinal tracts
B_1	Aids enzymes in breaking down and using carbohydrates; helps the nerves, muscles, and heart function efficiently
B_2	Aids enzymes in metabolism of fats and proteins
B_6	Aids enzymes in synthesis of amino acids
B_{12}	Works with folate in nucleic acid synthesis and metabolism of amino acids; coenzyme in metabolism of fatty acids
Folic acid	Works with cobalamins in nucleic acid synthesis and metabolism of amino acids; maintains red blood cells
C	Coenzyme involved in collagen production, capillary integrity, use of iron in hemoglobin, and synthesis of many hormones; improves absorption of iron; is an antioxidant
D	Builds bones and teeth; helps maintain calcium-phosphorus balance in blood
E	Aids in formation of red blood cells; maintains cell structure; is an intracellular antioxidant
K	Aids in blood clotting and bone growth

Source: Reprinted courtesy of the US Department of Agriculture.

Patient Education

Breast Self-Exam (BSE)

PATIENT EDUCATION TIPS

1. Explain the purpose of BSE.
2. Assist the patient to the standing position, and instruct her to use a large mirror to view the breasts during this part of the procedure.
3. Explain to the patient what she should look for when inspecting her breasts while standing.
4. Demonstrate the positioning of arms and hands for this visual inspection: first, her arms at her sides; then, her arms raised and her hands clasped behind her head; finally, her arms lowered with her hands on her hips.
5. Demonstrate, on the patient's breast, how to perform the small, rotary motions with the flat pads of the fingers from the outer rim (including the armpit and collarbone area) toward the nipple. (Synthetic breast models are available that may be helpful in teaching the proper technique.)
6. Demonstrate how to inspect the nipples.
7. Ask the patient to practice the procedure.
8. Observe the patient's self-exam technique. (If the patient is reluctant to examine herself in front of you, have her repeat the highlights of the procedure or use the synthetic model.)
9. Assist the patient to lie down with a small pillow or folded towel under the shoulder on the side to be examined.
10. Repeat steps 5 through 8.

11. Suggest that the patient mark her calendar for a monthly reminder to perform the exam 1 week after the onset of menses.
12. Give the patient educational materials that explain how to perform BSE.

Testicular Self-Exam (TSE)

PATIENT EDUCATION TIPS

1. TSE should be performed after a warm shower or bath, when scrotal skin is relaxed.
2. The man first observes the testes for changes in appearance, such as swelling. Hold the penis out of the way then manually examines each testicle, gently rolling it between the fingers and thumbs of both hands to feel for hard lumps.
3. The man should locate the area of the epididymis and spermatic cord and know these are normal structures. This area can be felt as a cord-like structure originating at the top back of each testicle.

Warning Signs of Cancer (*CAUTION*)

- **C**hange in bowel or bladder habits
- **A** sore that does not heal
- **U**nusual bleeding or discharge
- **T**hickening or lump in a breast or elsewhere
- **I**ndigestion or difficulty in swallowing
- **O**bvious change in a wart or mole
- **N**agging cough or hoarseness

Patient Instructions

Informing the Patient of Guidelines for Surgery

CRITICAL PROCEDURE STEPS

1. Review the patient's chart to determine the type of surgery to be performed.
2. Tell the patient that you will be providing both verbal and written instructions that should be followed prior to surgery.
3. Inform the patient about policies regarding makeup, jewelry, contact lenses, wigs, dentures, and so on.
4. Tell the patient to leave money and valuables at home.
5. If applicable, suggest appropriate clothing for the patient to wear for postoperative ease and comfort.
6. Explain the need for someone to drive the patient home following an outpatient surgical procedure.
7. Tell the patient the correct time to arrive in the office, surgery center, or hospital for the procedure.
8. Inform the patient of dietary restrictions. Be sure to use specific, clear instructions about what may or may not be ingested and at what time the patient must abstain from eating or drinking. Also explain these points:
   a. The reasons for the dietary restrictions
   b. The possible consequences of not following the dietary restrictions

continued

9. Ask patients who smoke to refrain from or reduce cigarette smoking during at least the 8 hours prior to the procedure. Explain to the patient that reducing smoking improves the level of oxygen in the blood during surgery.
10. Suggest that the patient shower or bathe the morning of the procedure or the evening before.
11. Instruct the patient about medications to take or avoid before surgery.
12. If necessary, clarify any information about which the patient is unclear.
13. Provide written surgical guidelines, and suggest that the patient call the office if additional questions arise.
14. Document the instruction in the patient's chart.

Pre-Exam Instructions

- Have the patient empty his bladder or bowels. (Collect a urine specimen if it is ordered.)
- Find out whether the patient has followed presurgical instructions.
- Measure the patient's vital signs.
- Ask if there are any symptoms or problems the physician should know about before surgery.
- Check the chart for ordered medications, such as pain medications or a tranquilizer.
- Ask the patient to disrobe according to the type of exam.
- Have the patient put on a gown and drape as indicated.

Post-Exam Instructions

- Administer postoperative medications.
- Ensure that the patient remains lying down for the prescribed length of time.

- Monitor the patient's vital signs.
- Watch for adverse reactions.
- Ask the patient to dress, and assist as necessary.
- Tell the patient when he might expect the results of any lab tests performed.
- Inform the patient if and when a follow-up appointment is needed.
- Document your observations.

Physical Exam

Assisting with a General PE

CRITICAL PROCEDURE STEPS

1. Wash your hands and adhere to standard precautions.
2. Assemble the equipment and supplies.
3. Arrange the equipment and supplies in a logical order for the physician's use.
4. Identify the patient.
5. Review the patient's medical history with the patient if required by office policy.
6. Obtain vital statistics.
7. Obtain the patient's weight and height.
8. Obtain a urine specimen before the patient undresses for the exam.
9. Explain the procedure and exam to the patient.
10. Obtain blood specimens or other laboratory tests as ordered.
11. Provide the patient with an appropriate gown and drape, and explain where the opening for the gown is placed.

continued

12. Obtain the ECG, if ordered.
13. Assist the patient to a sitting position at the end of the table with the drape placed across his legs.
14. Inform the physician that the patient is ready, and remain in the room to assist the physician.
15. You may be asked to shut off the light in the exam room to allow the patient's pupils to dilate for a retinal exam.
16. Hand the instruments to the physician as requested.
17. Assist the patient to the supine position for examination of the front of the body.
18. If a gynecologic exam is indicated, assist and drape the patient in the lithotomy position.
19. If a rectal exam is needed, assist and drape the patient in the Sims' position.
20. Assist the patient to a prone position for a posterior body examination.
21. When the exam is complete, assist the patient into the sitting position and have him sit for a brief period of time.
22. Ask the patient if he needs assistance in dressing.
23. Properly dispose of contaminated materials.
24. Remove the table paper and pillow covering, and dispose of them in the proper container.
25. Disinfect and clean counters and the table with a disinfectant.
26. Sanitize and sterilize instruments, if needed.
27. Prepare the room for the next patient by replacing the table paper, pillow cover, equipment, and supplies.
28. Document the procedure.

Assisting with a Needle Biopsy

CRITICAL PROCEDURE STEPS

1. Identify the patient and introduce yourself; instruct the patient as needed.

2. Wash your hands and assemble the necessary materials.

3. Prepare the sterile field and instruments.

4. Put on exam gloves.

5. Position the patient and cleanse the biopsy site. Prepare the patient's skin.

6. Remove the gloves, wash your hands, and put on clean exam gloves.

7. Assist the licensed practitioner as she injects anesthetic.

8. During the procedure, help drape and position the patient.

9. If you will be handing the practitioner the instruments, remove the gloves, perform a surgical scrub, and put on sterile gloves.

10. Place the sample in a properly labeled specimen bottle, complete the laboratory requisition form, and package the specimen for immediate transport to the laboratory.

11. Dress the patient's wound site.

12. Properly dispose of used supplies and instruments.

13. Clean and disinfect the room according to OSHA guidelines.

14. Remove the gloves and wash your hands.

15. Document as needed.

Components and Materials for a General Physical Exam

Component	Materials Required*
General appearance	No special materials
Head	No special materials
Neck	No special materials
Eyes and vision	Penlight, ophthalmoscope, vision and color vision charts
Ears and hearing	Otoscope, audiometer
Nose and sinuses	Penlight, nasal speculum
Mouth and throat	Gloves, tongue depressor
Chest and lungs	Stethoscope
Heart	Stethoscope
Breasts	No special materials
Abdomen	Stethoscope
Genitalia (women)	Gloves, vaginal speculum, lubricant
Genitalia (men)	Gloves
Rectum	Gloves, lubricant
Musculoskeletal system	Tape measure
Neurologic system	Reflex hammer, penlight

*Gloves should always be worn if your hands will come in contact with the patient's nonintact skin, blood, and/or body fluids.

Exam Methods (Common Order of Performance)

Inspection

- The visualization of the patient's entire body and overall appearance

- Used to assess posture, mannerisms, hygiene, body size, shape, color, position, symmetry, and the presence of rashes or growths

Auscultation

- The process of listening to body sounds
- Used to assess sounds from the heart, lungs, and abdominal organs

Palpation

- The process of using touch to assess a patient's body parts
- Used to assess texture, temperature, shape, and the presence of vibrations or movement in underlying tissues

Percussion

- Tapping or striking the body to hear sounds or feel vibrations
- Used to determine the location, size, or density of a body structure or organ under the skin

Mensuration

- The process of measuring
- Used to assess height and weight, growth, and extremity or wound diameter

Manipulation

- The systematic moving of a patient's body parts
- Used to check for abnormalities that affect movement

Positions

Sitting

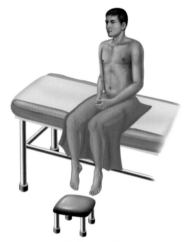

Sitting position

- The patient sits at the edge of the examining table without back support.
- The physician examines the patient's head, neck, chest, heart, back, and arms.
- While the patient is in the sitting position, the physician evaluates the patient's ability to fully expand the lungs.
- She then checks the upper body parts for symmetry, the degree to which one side is the same as the other.

- In this position the drape is placed across the patient's lap for men or across the patient's chest and lap for women.
- If a patient is too weak to sit unsupported, another position is necessary. One possible alternative is the supine position.

Supine (recumbent)

- The patient lies flat on the back.
- This is the most relaxed position for many patients.
- A doctor can examine the head, neck, chest, heart, abdomen, arms, and legs when a patient is in the supine position.
- The patient is normally draped from the neck or underarms down to the feet.
- The supine position may not be comfortable for patients who become short of breath easily. Also, patients with a back injury or lower-back pain may find it uncomfortable.
- You can make these patients more comfortable by placing a pillow under their heads and under their knees. Some patients, however, may need to be placed in the dorsal recumbent position.

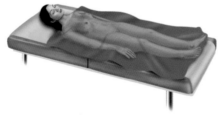

Supine position

Dorsal recumbent

- The patient lies face up, with his back supporting all his weight.
- This position is the same as the supine position, except that the patient's knees are drawn up and the feet are flat on the table.
- The physician may examine the head, neck, chest, and heart while a patient is in this position.
- The patient is normally draped from the neck or underarms down to the feet.
- Patients who have leg disabilities may find the dorsal recumbent position uncomfortable or even impossible.
- Patients who are elderly or have painful disorders such as arthritis or back pain may find the dorsal recumbent position more comfortable than the supine position because the knees are bent.
- This position is sometimes used as an alternative to the lithotomy position when patients have severe arthritis or joint deformities.

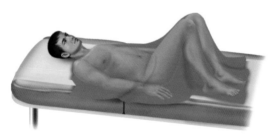

Dorsal recumbent position

Fowler's

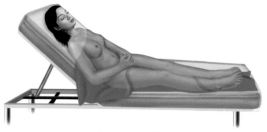

Fowler's position

- The patient lies back on an examining table on which the head is elevated.
- The head of the table can be raised to a 90-degree angle; the most common position is a 45-degree angle.
- The doctor may examine the head, neck, and chest areas while the patient is in this position.
- The patient is usually draped from the neck or underarms down to the feet.
- Fowler's position is one of the best positions for examining patients who are experiencing shortness of breath or individuals with a lower-back injury.

Knee-elbow (knee-chest)

- The patient lies on the table facedown, supporting the body with the knees and elbows or chest.
- The patient should have the thighs at a 90-degree angle to the table and slightly separated.
- The head is turned to one side, and the arms are placed to the side or above the head.
- The patient may need your assistance to assume this position correctly and to maintain it during the exam.

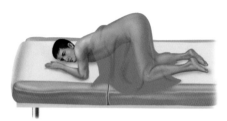

Knee-chest position

- The knee-elbow or -chest position is used during exams of the anal and perineal areas and during certain proctologic procedures.
- Some patients—those who are pregnant, obese, or elderly—have difficulty assuming the knee-chest position. The knee-elbow position puts less strain on the patient and is easier to maintain. The knee-elbow position supports body weight with the knees and elbows rather than the knees and chest.
- In either of these two positions, the patient is commonly covered with a fenestrated drape, in which a special opening provides access to the area to be examined.

Lithotomy

- The patient lies on her back with her knees bent and her feet in stirrups attached to the end of the examining table.
- You may need to help the patient place her feet in the stirrups. She should then slide forward to position her buttocks near the edge of the table.
- Many women are embarrassed and physically uncomfortable in this position, so you should not ask a patient to remain in this position any longer than necessary.

162

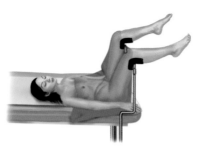

Lithotomy position

- Use a large drape that covers the patient from the breasts to the ankles. Placing the drape with one point or corner between the legs will make the exam easier in this position.
- A patient with severe arthritis or joint deformities in the hips or knees may have difficulty assuming the lithotomy position. She may be able to place only one leg in the stirrup, or she may need your assistance in separating her thighs.
- An alternative position for such a patient is the dorsal recumbent position. Other patients who may have difficulty with the lithotomy position are those who are obese or in the late stages of pregnancy.

Proctologic

- The patient is bent at the hips at a 90-degree angle.
- The patient can assume this position by standing next to the examining table and bending at the waist until the chest rests on the table.
- If an adjustable examining table is available, the patient can assume the position by lying prone on the table, which is then raised in the middle with both ends

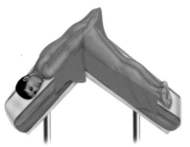

Proctologic position

pointing down. This places the patient at the correct 90-degree angle.

- In either variation of this position, the patient is draped with a fenestrated drape, as in the knee-elbow position.

Prone

- The patient lies flat on the table, facedown.
- The patient's head is turned to one side, and his arms are placed at his sides or bent at the elbows.
- The patient is normally draped from the upper back to the feet.
- With the patient in this position, the physician can examine the back, feet, or musculoskeletal system.
- The prone position is unsuitable for women in advanced stages of pregnancy, obese patients, patients with respiratory difficulties, and the elderly.

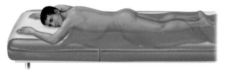

Prone position

Sims'

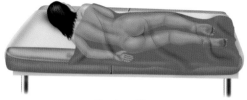

Sims' position

- The patient lies on the left side with the left leg slightly bent, and the left arm placed behind the back so that the patient's weight is resting primarily on the chest.
- The right knee is bent and raised toward the chest, and the right arm is bent toward the head for support.
- The patient is draped from the upper back to the feet.
- Sims' position is used during anal or rectal exams and may be used for perineal and certain pelvic exams.
- Patients with joint deformities of the hips and knees may have difficulty assuming this position.

Positioning the Patient for an Exam

CRITICAL PROCEDURE STEPS

1. Identify the patient and introduce yourself.
2. Wash your hands.
3. Explain the procedure to the patient.
4. Provide a gown or drape if the physician has requested one, and instruct the patient in the proper way to wear it after disrobing. Allow the patient privacy while disrobing, and assist only if the patient requests help.

continued

5. Explain to the patient the necessary exam and the position required.

6. Ask the patient to step on the stool or the pullout step of the examining table. If necessary, assist the patient onto the examining table.

7. Assist the patient into the required position.

8. Drape the patient to prevent exposure and avoid embarrassment. Place pillows for comfort as needed.

9. Adjust the drapes during the exam.

10. On completion of the exam, assist the patient as necessary out of the position and provide privacy as the client dresses.

Vision Screening

CRITICAL PROCEDURE STEPS

Distance Vision

1. Wash your hands, clean the occluder, identify the patient, and explain the procedure.

2. Mount the eye chart at eye level.

3. Make a mark on the floor 20 feet away from the chart.

4. Have the patient stand at the 20-foot mark with her heels at the line.

5. Instruct the patient to keep both eyes open and not to squint or lean forward during the test.

6. Test the patient's eyes in order according to office policy.

7. Have the patient read the lines beginning with the 20-foot line or according to office policy.
8. Note the smallest line the patient can read or identify.
9. Record the results as a fraction.
10. Repeat the procedure for each eye.
11. Record the results for each eye.
12. Note and record any observations of squinting, head tilting, or excessive blinking or tearing.
13. Ask the patient to keep both eyes open and to identify the color of the two colored bars on the Snellen chart, and record the results.
14. Clean the occluder with a gauze square dampened with alcohol.
15. Properly dispose of the gauze square and wash your hands.

Near Vision

1. Wash your hands, identify the patient, and explain the procedure.
2. Have the patient hold the near vision card at a distance of 14 to 16 inches.
3. Have the patient keep both eyes open and read or identify the letters, symbols, or paragraphs.
4. Record the smallest line read without error.
5. Clean the card if indicated.
6. Wash your hands.

Color Vision

1. Wash your hands, identify the patient, and explain the procedure.
2. Hold one of the color charts or books at the patient's normal reading distance.

continued

3. Ask the patient to tell you the number or symbol within the colored dots on each chart or page.
4. Proceed through all the charts or pages.
5. Record the number correctly identified and failed with a slash between them.
6. Clean the charts if indicated.
7. Wash your hands.
8. Document the procedure.

Pulmonary Function

Respiratory Air Volumes, Capacities, and Tests

Name	Volume*	Description
Tidal volume (TV)	500 mL	Volume moved into or out of the lungs during a respiratory cycle
Inspiratory reserve volume (IRV)	3,000 mL	Volume that can be inhaled during forced breathing in addition to resting tidal volume
Expiratory reserve volume (ERV)	1,100 mL	Volume that can be exhaled during forced breathing in addition to resting tidal volume
Residual volume (RV)	1,200 mL	Volume that remains in the lungs at all times

Name	Volume*	Description
Inspiratory capacity (IC)	3,500 mL	Maximum volume of air that can be inhaled following exhalation of resting tidal volume: IC = TV + IRV
Functional residual capacity (FRC)	2,300 mL	Volume of air that remains in the lungs following exhalation of resting tidal volume: FRC = ERV + RV
Vital capacity	4,600 mL	Maximum volume of air that can be exhaled after taking the deepest breath possible: VC = TV + IRV + ERV
Total lung capacity (TLC)	5,800 mL	Total volume of air that the lungs can hold: TLC = VC + RV
Forced vital capacity (FVC)	Varies depending on gender, age, and height	Amount of air exhaled with force after inhaling as deeply as possible
Peak expiratory flow (PEF)	Varies depending on gender, age, and height	Greatest rate of flow during forced exhalation

*Values are typical for a tall, young adult.

Vital Signs and Measurements

Apical Pulse

Location

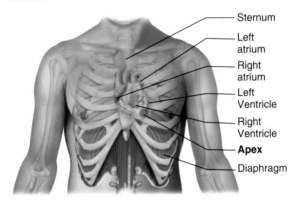

Blood Pressure (BP)

Taking BP of adults and older children

CRITICAL PROCEDURE STEPS

1. Gather the equipment and make sure it is in working order and calibrated.
2. Identify the patient.
3. Wash your hands and explain the procedure.
4. Have the patient sit in a quiet area and roll up her sleeves if indicated.

5. Have the patient rest her arm on a flat surface so that the midpoint of the upper arm is at heart level.

6. Select an appropriate-sized cuff.

7. Locate the brachial artery.

8. Position the cuff so that the midline of the bladder is above the arterial pulsation, 1 inch above the antecubital space.

9. Place the manometer's dial at eye level so that it can be easily read.

10. Close the valve of the pressure bulb until it is finger tight.

11. Inflate the cuff rapidly to 70 mm Hg, then in 10-mm Hg increments while palpating the radial pulse with your other hand.

12. Note the level of pressure where the radial pulse disappears and subsequently reappears when the pressure is released.

13. Open the valve, release the pressure completely, and wait at least 30 seconds.

14. Place the stethoscope earpieces in your ears, adjusting for comfort and a snug fit.

15. Place the head of the stethoscope over the brachial artery pulsation, holding it firmly in place with the index and middle fingers.

16. Inflate the bladder rapidly to 30 mm Hg above the palpated pressure.

17. Open the valve and slowly deflate the cuff 2 mm Hg per second.

18. As the pressure falls, note the level of pressure where the first repetitive sounds appear (systolic pressure).

continued

19. Continue deflating the cuff and note the point at which the sound changes from strong to muffled.

20. Continue deflating the cuff and note when the sound disappears (diastolic pressure).

21. Deflate the cuff completely and remove it from the patient's arm.

22. Record the systolic and diastolic numbers, separated by a slash, in the patient's chart.

23. Properly store the cuff in the holder.

24. Disinfect the earpieces and diaphragm of the stethoscope with alcohol.

25. Properly dispose of any disposable supplies.

26. Wash your hands.

Taking BP of a young child

CRITICAL PROCEDURE STEPS

1. Ideally, take the patient's blood pressure before performing other tests or procedures that may cause anxiety. In this way, you can avoid a falsely high result.

2. Be sure to use the correct cuff size for the child or infant. The bladder width should not exceed two-thirds the length of the upper or lower arm. The bladder should cover three-fourths the circumference of the extremity.

3. Do not attempt to estimate an infant's blood pressure by the palpatory method.

4. Inflate the pressure cuff to 20 mm Hg above the point at which the radial pulse disappears.
5. Deflate the cuff at a rate of 2 mm Hg per second.
6. You may continue to hear a pulse beat on a child or an infant until the pressure reaches zero, so note when the strong pulse beat becomes muffled.

Conversions and Equivalents

Height

In	Cm	In	Cm	In	Cm
20	51	42	107	64	163
22	56	44	112	66	168
24	61	46	117	68	173
26	66	48	122	70	178
28	71	50	127	72	183
30	76	52	132	74	188
32	81	54	137	76	193
34	86	56	142	78	198
36	91	58	147	80	203
38	97	60	152		
40	102	62	157		

Note: cm = in × 2.54. Conversions are rounded to nearest whole number.

Temperature

°F	°C	°F	°C	°F	°C
95.0	35.0	99.4	37.4	103.8	39.9
95.2	35.1	99.6	37.6	104.0	40.0
95.4	35.2	99.8	37.7	104.2	40.1
95.6	35.3	100.0	37.8	104.4	40.2
95.8	35.4	100.2	37.9	104.6	40.3
96.0	35.6	100.4	38.0	104.8	40.4
96.2	35.7	100.6	38.1	105.0	40.6
96.4	35.8	100.8	38.2	105.2	40.7
96.6	35.9	101.0	38.3	105.4	40.8
96.8	36.0	101.2	38.4	105.6	40.9
97.0	36.1	101.4	38.6	105.8	41.0
97.2	36.2	101.6	38.7	106.0	41.1
97.4	36.3	101.8	38.8	106.2	41.2
97.6	36.4	102.0	38.9	106.4	41.3
97.8	36.6	102.2	39.0	106.6	41.4
98.0	36.7	102.4	39.1	106.8	41.6
98.2	36.8	102.6	39.2	107.0	41.7
98.4	36.9	102.8	39.3	107.2	41.8
98.6	37.0	103.0	39.4	107.4	41.9
98.8	37.1	103.2	39.6	107.6	42.0
99.0	37.2	103.4	39.7	107.8	42.1
99.2	37.3	103.6	39.8	108.0	42.2

Weight

Lb	Kg	Lb	Kg	Lb	Kg
10	4.5	95	43.1	180	81.7
15	6.8	100	45.4	185	84.0
20	9.1	105	47.7	190	86.3
25	11.4	110	49.9	195	88.5
30	13.6	115	52.2	200	90.8
35	15.9	120	54.5	205	93.1
40	18.2	125	56.8	210	95.3
45	20.4	130	59.0	215	97.6
50	22.7	135	61.3	220	99.9
55	25.0	140	63.6	225	102.2
60	27.2	145	65.8	230	104.4
65	29.5	150	68.1	235	106.7
70	31.8	155	70.4	240	109.0
75	34.1	160	72.6	245	111.2
80	36.3	165	74.9	250	113.5
85	38.6	170	77.2		
90	40.9	175	79.5		

Note: kg = lb × 0.454; lb = kg × 2.205. Conversions are rounded to nearest tenth.

Measuring Height

Adults and older children

CRITICAL PROCEDURE STEPS

1. With the patient off the scale, raise the height bar well above the patient's head and swing out the extension.
2. Ask the patient to step on the center of the scale and to stand up straight and look forward.
3. Gently lower the height bar until the extension rests on the patient's head.
4. Have the patient step off the scale before reading the measurement.
5. If the patient is less than 50 inches tall, read the height on the bottom part of the ruler; if the patient is more than 50 inches tall, read the height on the top, movable part of the ruler at the point at which it meets the bottom part of the ruler. Note that the numbers increase on the bottom part of the bar and decrease on the top, movable part of the bar. Read the height in the right direction.
6. Record the patient's height.
7. Have the patient put her shoes back on, if necessary.
8. Properly dispose of the towel (if used) and wash your hands.

CRITICAL PROCEDURE STEPS

1. Measure the child's height in the same manner as you measure adult height, or have the child stand with his back against the height chart. Measure height at the crown of the head.
2. Record the height in the patient's chart.
3. Properly dispose of the towel (if used) and wash your hands.

Measuring Weight

Adults and older children

CRITICAL PROCEDURE STEPS

1. Identify the patient and introduce yourself.
2. Wash your hands and explain the procedure to the patient.
3. Check to see whether the scale is in balance by moving all the weights to the left side. The indicator should be level with the middle mark. If not, check the manufacturer's directions and adjust it to ensure a zero balance. If you are using a scale equipped to measure either kilograms or pounds, check to see that it is set on the desired units and that the upper and lower weights show the same units.
4. Ask the patient to remove her shoes, if that is the standard office policy.

continued

5. Place a disposable towel on the scale or have the patient leave her socks on.

6. Ask the patient to step on the center of the scale, facing forward. Assist as necessary.

7. Place the lower weight at the highest number that does not cause the balance indicator to drop to the bottom.

8. Move the upper weight slowly to the right until the balance bar is centered at the middle mark, adjusting as necessary.

9. Add the two weights together to get the patient's weight.

10. Record the patient's weight in the chart to the nearest quarter of a pound or tenth of a kilogram.

11. Return the weights to their starting positions on the left side.

Toddlers

CRITICAL PROCEDURE STEPS

1. Identify the patient and obtain permission from the parent to weigh the toddler.

2. Wash your hands and explain the procedure to the parent.

3. Check to see whether the scale is in balance, and place a disposable towel on the scale or have the patient wear shoes or socks, depending upon the policy of the facility.

4. Ask the parent to hold the patient and to step on the scale. Follow the procedure for obtaining the weight of an adult.

5. Have the parent put the child down or hand the child to another staff member.

6. Obtain the parent's weight.

7. Subtract the parent's weight from the combined weight to determine the weight of the child.

8. Record the patient's weight in the chart to the nearest quarter of a pound or tenth of a kilogram.

Measuring Infants

CRITICAL PROCEDURE STEPS

Weight

1. Identify the patient and obtain permission from the parent to weigh the infant.

2. Wash your hands and explain the procedure to the parent.

3. Ask the parent to undress the infant.

4. Place the disposable towel on the infant scale; then check to see whether it is in balance.

5. Have the parent place the child face up on the scale (or on the examining table if the scale is built into it). Keep one hand over the infant at all times and hold a diaper over a male patient's penis to catch any urine the infant might void.

continued

6. Place the lower weight at the highest number that does not cause the balance indicator to drop to the bottom.

7. Move the upper weight slowly to the right until the balance bar is centered at the middle mark, adjusting as necessary.

8. Add the two weights together to get the infant's weight.

9. Record the infant's weight in the chart in pounds and ounces or to the nearest tenth of a kilogram.

10. Return the weights to their starting positions on the left side.

Length: Scale with Length (Height) Bar

11. If the scale has a height bar, move the infant toward the head of the scale or examining table until her head touches the bar.

12. Have the parent hold the infant by the shoulders in this position.

13. Holding the infant's ankles, gently extend the legs and slide the bottom bar to touch the soles of the feet.

14. Note the length and release the infant's ankles.

15. Record the length in the patient's chart.

Length: Scale or Examining Table Without Length (Height) Bar

16. If neither the scale nor the examining table has a height bar, have the parent position the infant close to the head of the examining table and hold the infant by the shoulders in this position.

17. Place a stiff piece of cardboard against the crown of the infant's head, and mark a line on the towel or paper, or hold a yardstick against the cardboard.

18. Holding the infant's ankles, gently extend the legs and draw a line on the towel or paper to mark the heel, or note the measure on the yardstick.

19. Release the infant's ankles and measure the distance between the two markings on the towel or paper using the yardstick or a tape measure.

20. Record the length in the patient's chart or on the growth chart.

Head Circumference

21. With the infant in a sitting or supine position, place the tape measure around the infant's head at the forehead.

22. Adjust the tape so that it surrounds the infant's head at its largest circumference.

23. Overlap the ends of the tape, and read the measure at the point of overlap.

24. Remove the tape, and record the circumference in the patient's chart.

25. Properly dispose of the used towel and wash your hands.

Normal Ranges for Vital Signs

Vital Sign	Age					
	0–1 Year	1–2 Years	2–5 Years	6–12 Years	Greater Than 12 Years	Adult
Temperature						
• Oral (°F)		97.9–100.4	97.9–100.4	95.9–99.5	97.6–99.6	97.8–99.1
• Rectal (°F)	99–100	97.9–100.4	97.9–100.4	97.9–100.4	98.6–100.6	98.8–100.1
Pulse (beats per minute)	100–160	90–150	80–140	70–120	60–100	60–100
Respirations (per minute)	30–60	24–40	22–34	18–30	12–16	12–18
Blood pressure (mm Hg)*						
• Systolic	80–114	84–117	85–123	91–135	104–147	Less than 120
• Diastolic	34–67	39–72	44–82	53–91	60–97	Less than 80

Note: Normal vital signs vary. Always compare your results with previous results obtained on the patient.

*Classifications for adult blood pressure are seen in the following table. Pediatric blood pressure ranges vary greatly based on height percentiles and gender. Always consult the physician regarding specific ranges for each patient.

Blood Pressure Classifications

Classification	Systolic (mm Hg)	Diastolic (mm Hg)
Normal	Less than 120	AND/OR less than 80
Prehypertension	120–139	AND/OR 80–89
Stage 1 hypertension	140–159	AND/OR 90–99
Stage 2 hypertension	Greater than 160	AND/OR greater than 100

Pulse

Characteristics

- **Rhythm**—may be regular or irregular
- **Volume**—may be weak, strong, or bounding

Pulse volume

- 0 = No palpable pulse
- 1+ = Weak
- 2+ = Faint pulse
- 3+ = Normal pulse
- 4+ = Bounding pulse

Locations

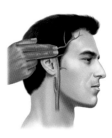

Temporal artery

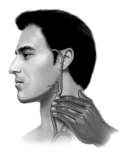

Carotid artery

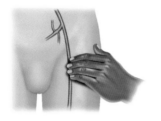

Femoral artery

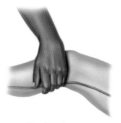

Popliteal artery

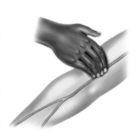

Brachial artery

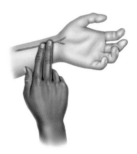

Radial artery

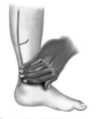

Posterior tibial artery

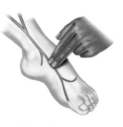

Dorsalis pedis artery

CRITICAL PROCEDURE STEPS

1. Gather the equipment and wash your hands.
2. Identify the patient.
3. Explain the procedure but do not say you are counting respirations.
4. Place the patient in a comfortable position with her arm resting on the table, palm down.
5. Position yourself so you can observe or feel the chest wall movements.
6. Locate the radial pulse and place two or three fingers on it.
7. Count the pulse for 30 seconds if regular and 1 full minute if irregular.
8. Without letting go of the wrist, count the respirations for 1 full minute.
9. Record the pulse and respirations.
10. Document results with the date and time.
11. Report any numbers that are a significant change or outside the range.

Vitamins and Minerals

1. Beta carotene
   - Megadose—more than 1.5 to 1.8 mg
   - Claims/benefits—improves the body's chemical reactions to dangerous free radicals, with health-promoting effects such as preventing lung cancer or heart disease for ex-smokers

- Possible health hazard—lung cancer, death, headache, vomiting, joint pain, hair loss, jaundice, liver damage

2. Folic acid
   - Megadose—more than 1,000 mg
   - Claims/benefits—reduces the risk of heart disease
   - Possible health hazard—no known adverse effects

3. Niacin
   - Megadose—slow-release doses of 500 mg or more or immediate-release doses of 750 mg or more
   - Claims/benefits—decreases cholesterol
   - Possible health hazard—stomach pain, vomiting, bloating, nausea, cramping, diarrhea, liver disease, muscle disease, eye damage, blood vessel dilation, hypotension, heart injury

4. Selenium
   - Megadose—800 to 1,000 micrograms
   - Claims/benefits—reduces cancer risk
   - Possible health hazard—tissue damage of the hair, nails, liver, nervous system, and teeth

5. Vitamin A
   - Megadose—25,000 or more international units
   - Claims/benefits—antioxidant that protects cells from free radicals that can cause chronic diseases
   - Possible health hazard—birth defects, bone abnormalities, severe liver disease

6. Vitamin B_6
   - Megadose—more than 100 mg

- Claims/benefits—treats asthma and cardiovascular disease
- Possible health hazard—balance difficulties, nerve injury causing changes in touch sensation

7. Vitamin C
   - Megadose—more than 100 mg
   - Claims/benefits—improves the body's chemical reactions to dangerous free radicals, with health-promoting effects such as preventing lung cancer or heart disease for ex-smokers
   - Possible health hazard—gastrointestinal distress and kidney stones

8. Vitamin D
   - Megadose—more than 2.5 mg
   - Claims/benefits—treats tuberculosis, rheumatoid arthritis, and skin disorders
   - Possible health hazard—bone demineralization, tendonitis, skeletal pain, potential heart and kidney damage

9. Vitamin E
   - Megadose—more than 400 to 1,000 international units
   - Claims/benefits—improves the body's chemical reactions to dangerous free radicals, with health-promoting effects such as preventing lung cancer or heart disease for ex-smokers
   - Possible health hazard—increased blood coagulation, stroke, death

3 Laboratory

Blood Tests

Blood Draw Order and Tube Additives

When drawing multiple tubes of blood, you should collect them in the order listed below. This reduces the chance of cross-contaminating the tube additives.

Stopper Color	Additive
Yellow	Sodium polyanethol sulfonate
Light blue	Sodium citrate
Red	• Clot activator • Silicone-coated
Gold or red/gray	• Clot activator • Silicone serum separator
Green	Heparin
Lavender	Ethylenediaminetetraacetic acid (EDTA) (anticoagulant)
Gray	Potassium oxalate or sodium fluoride (anticoagulant)

Preparing a Blood Smear

CRITICAL PROCEDURE STEPS

1. Wash your hands and put on exam gloves.

2. If you will be using blood from a capillary puncture, express a drop of blood from the patient's finger. If you will be using a venous specimen, check the specimen for proper labeling, carefully uncap the specimen tube, and use wooden applicator sticks to remove any coagulated blood from the inside rim of the tube. You may use a safety transfer device if available.

3. Touch the tip of the capillary tube to the blood specimen from either the patient's finger or the specimen tube. The tube will take up the correct amount through capillary action.

4. Pull the capillary tube away from the specimen, holding it carefully to prevent spillage. Wipe the outside of the capillary tube with a sterile gauze square.

5. With the slide on the work surface, hold the capillary tube in one hand and the frosted end of the slide against the work surface with the other.

6. Apply a drop of blood to the slide, about ¾ inch from the frosted end. Place the capillary tube in the sharps container.

7. Pick up the spreader slide with your dominant hand. Hold the slide at approximately a 30- to 35-degree angle. Place the edge of the spreader slide on the smear slide close to the unfrosted end. Pull the spreader slide toward the frosted end until the spreader slide touches the blood drop. Capillary action will spread the droplet along the edge of the spreader slide.

8. As soon as the drop spreads out to cover most of the spreader slide edge, push the spreader slide back toward the unfrosted end of the smear slide, pulling the specimen across the slide behind it. Maintain the 30- to 35-degree angle.

9. Continue pushing until the spreader slide comes off the end, still maintaining the angle. The resulting smear should be approximately 1½ inches long, preferably with a margin of empty slide on all sides. The smear should be thicker on the frosted end of the slide.

10. Properly label the slide, allow it to dry, and follow the manufacturer's directions for staining it for the required tests.

11. Properly dispose of used supplies and disinfect the work area.

12. Remove the gloves and wash your hands.

Quality Control for Specimen Collection

CRITICAL PROCEDURE STEPS

1. Review the requisition form for the test ordered and verify the procedure.

2. Prepare the equipment, paperwork, and work area.

3. Identify the patient and explain the procedure.

4. Confirm that the patient has followed any pretest preparation requirements.

5. Collect the specimen properly.

continued

6. Use the correct specimen collection containers and the right additives, if required.
7. Immediately label the specimens.
8. Follow correct procedure for disposing of biohazardous waste and decontaminating the work area.
9. Thank the patient, and keep the patient in the office for follow-up observation if required.
10. Properly prepare the specimen for transport to an outside lab if indicated.

YOU SHOULD KNOW

Causes of Lab Errors

- Improperly calibrated equipment
- Reagents out of date
- Contaminated reagents
- Controls not done or improperly done
- Improperly performed testing procedure
- Incorrect timing
- Improperly collected sample
- Incorrect interpretation of results

Common Lab Tests (Waived Tests)

| Urine tests | Urinalysis by dipstick (reagent strip) or tablet reagent (nonautomated) for bilirubin, glucose, hemoglobin, ketone, leukocytes, nitrite, pH, protein, specific gravity, and urobilinogen |

Urine tests (cont.)	Ovulation (visual color comparison tests)
	Pregnancy (visual color comparison tests)
	Home-screening tests for drugs (opioids, cocaine, methamphetamines, cannabinoids)
	Nicotine detection tests
	Urine chemistry analyzer for microalbumin and creatinine (semi-quantitative)
	Tumor-associated antigen for bladder cancer (using devices approved by the FDA for home use)
	Catalase
Blood tests	Erythrocyte sedimentation rate (ESR), nonautomated
	Hemoglobin by copper sulfate, nonautomated
	Spun microhematocrit
	Blood glucose (using devices approved by the FDA for home use)
	Hemoglobin by single analyte instruments, automated
	Prothrombin time
	Ketones in whole blood, OTC test only
	Total cholesterol, HDL, LDL, and triglycerides
	Hemoglobin A1c
	Lactate in whole blood
	Lead in whole blood
	Thyroid-stimulating hormone, rapid test
	Mononucleosis rapid test
	Helicobacter pylori rapid antibody test

Source: Reprinted courtesy of the US Department of Health and Human Services.

Collection Techniques

Capillary Puncture

CRITICAL PROCEDURE STEPS

1. Review the laboratory requisition and gather the supplies.
2. Identify the patient.
3. Explain the procedure; confirm that the patient has followed the pretest procedures.
4. Position the patient in the venipuncture chair or lying down.
5. Wash your hands and put on gloves.
6. Examine the patient's hands to determine which finger to use (generally one of the middle two fingers). Warm the patient's hands if necessary.
7. Gently massage the finger.
8. Clean the area with antiseptic and allow to air-dry.
9. Hold the patient's finger between your thumb and forefinger.
10. Puncture the finger with the puncture device.
11. Allow a drop of blood to form at the end of the patient's finger.
12. Wipe away the first drop of blood.
13. Fill the collection device.
14. Dispose of the lancet.
15. Wipe the patient's finger with a sterile gauze square.
16. Have the patient apply pressure to the puncture site.
17. Label the specimen and complete the laboratory requisition form or perform the test.

18. Check the puncture site for bleeding.
19. Properly dispose of used supplies and disposable instruments.
20. Remove the gloves and wash your hands.
21. Instruct the patient about care of the puncture site.
22. Document the procedure and record the results if appropriate.

Venipuncture

CRITICAL PROCEDURE STEPS

1. Review the laboratory requisition form and gather the supplies.
2. Identify the patient.
3. Explain the procedure; confirm that the patient has followed the pretest procedures.
4. Position the patient in the venipuncture chair or lying down.
5. Wash your hands and put on gloves.
6. Insert the threaded end of the needle into the safety needle holder and push the first collection tube partway into the holder.
7. Position the patient's arm slightly downward.
8. Apply the tourniquet to the patient's upper arm midway between the elbow and shoulder.
9. Palpate the proposed site with your index finger to locate the vein.

continued

10. Clean the area with an antiseptic wipe, using a circular motion, and allow to air-dry.

11. Remove the plastic cap from the outer point of the needle, ask the patient to make a fist, and pull the skin taut below the insertion site.

12. Insert the needle at a 15-degree angle, bevel side up.

13. Seat the collection tube in place on the needle, puncturing the rubber stopper. Fill the tube(s).

14. Once blood flow is steady, have the patient release his fist; untie the tourniquet.

15. Withdraw the needle with a smooth, steady motion and place a sterile gauze square over the insertion site.

16. Immediately activate the safety device.

17. Ask the patient to hold pressure at the site.

18. Slowly invert the collection tubes if they contain additives.

19. Label the specimens and complete the paperwork.

20. Observe the patient's condition and check the site for bleeding.

21. Place a pressure dressing over the puncture site.

22. Properly dispose of used supplies and disposable instruments.

23. Remove the gloves and wash your hands.

24. Instruct the patient about when to remove the pressure dressing.

25. Document the procedure in the patient's chart.

Venipuncture Complications

Complication	Tips for Avoiding Complications
Hematoma	• Hold the needle as still as possible. • Use a butterfly system for small veins. • Hold pressure at the puncture site as soon as you remove the needle.
Infection	• Use only approved single-use equipment. • Clean the puncture site thoroughly.
Latex allergy	• Before the procedure, ask the patient if he has any allergies. • Use non-latex gloves, tourniquets, and bandages.
Nerve injury	Review the anatomy of the antecubital fossa prior to performing the procedure.

Special Considerations

- Children—address the child directly; speaking in a calm, soothing voice, briefly explain the procedure.
- Difficult venipuncture—if your first attempt fails, try another site. Ask for assistance after two attempts.
- Elderly patients—speak in low, clear tones. Take your time with the procedure.
- Fainting—position the patient in a venipuncture chair so that if he does faint, no injury will occur.
- Patients at risk for uncontrolled bleeding—be careful and alert, hold a cotton ball over the venipuncture site for at least 5 minutes, and alert the physician if bleeding does not stop after 5 minutes.

Labeled Microscope and Tips

Care and Cleaning

- Clean the microscope after each use.
- Inspect the body tube, arm, and stage for dust and other contaminants.
- Clean the oculars and lenses with lens paper, not tissue.
- Use lens cleaning products according to the manufacturer's guidelines.
- Store the microscope with the cover on and the cord wrapped loosely around the base.
- Carry the microscope with one hand on the arm and one supporting the base.

Identification

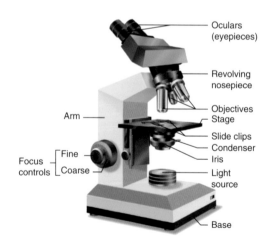

Oculars (eyepieces)

Revolving nosepiece

Objectives
Stage

Slide clips
Condenser
Iris

Light source

Arm

Focus controls — Fine
Focus controls — Coarse

Base

Using a Microscope

CRITICAL PROCEDURE STEPS

1. Wash your hands and put on gloves.
2. Examine the microscope to make sure it is clean and all parts are intact.
3. Plug in the microscope and make sure the light is working.
4. Turn the light off and clean the lenses with lens paper.
5. Place the specimen slide on the stage and secure it in place.
6. Position distance between the oculars to a position of comfort.
7. Adjust the 10× objective so that it points directly at the specimen, leaving enough space so that the slide does not touch the objective.
8. Turn on the light and adjust the iris so that light fills the field without washing it out.
9. Observe the slide from one side and adjust the body tube to move the objective closer to the specimen.
10. Use the coarse focus to slowly bring the image into focus.
11. Use the fine focus until the image is clearly visible.
12. Switch to the 40× objective and refocus using the fine focus.
13. Rotate the objective assembly so that no objective points at the specimen.
14. Add a drop of immersion oil to the slide.

continued

15. Rotate the 100× objective into the oil.
16. Examine the image and adjust the light and focus using the fine focus only as needed.
17. After examining the specimen, lower the stage and raise the objectives.
18. Remove the slide and dispose of it or store it.
19. Turn off the light and unplug the microscope according to office policy.
20. Carefully clean the stage, ocular lenses, and objectives, removing all traces of immersion oil.
21. Point the 10× objective toward the stage and lower it so that it is close to but not touching the stage.
22. Cover the microscope and clean the area.
23. Remove your gloves and wash your hands.

Lab Slip Completion

YOU SHOULD KNOW

When completing a laboratory requisition slip, you should include the following information:

- Patient's full name, sex, date of birth, medical record number, and address or location if an inpatient
- Patient's insurance information
- Ordering facility or provider
- Physician's name, address, and phone number
- Type of specimen and where and how it was collected
- Date and time of the specimen collection
- Test(s) requested, including status such as fasting
- Preliminary diagnosis
- Any current treatment that might affect the results

Microbiology Review

Classification of Microorganisms

- **Prions**—infectious particles made of protein
- **Bacteria**—single-celled, prokaryotic organisms
- **Fungi**—eukaryotic organisms with a rigid cell wall
- **Helminths**—multicellular parasites that live on or in another organism and use that other organism for their own nourishment, or for some other advantage, to the detriment of the host organism
- **Protozoans**—single-celled, eukaryotic organisms, usually larger than bacteria
- **Viruses**—consist of nucleic acid and a protein coat

Diagnosing and Treating Infections

The following are the basic steps:

- Examining the patient
- Obtaining specimens
- Examining the specimens directly
- Culturing the specimens
- Determining the culture's antibiotic sensitivity
- Treating the patient as ordered by the physician

Obtaining a Throat Culture

CRITICAL PROCEDURE STEPS

1. Identify the patient and explain the procedure.
2. Assemble the necessary supplies and label the culture plate if used.

continued

3. Wash your hands and don gloves, goggles, and a mask or face shield.

4. Have the patient assume a sitting position.

5. Open the collection system or swab package and remove the swab with your dominant hand.

6. Ask the patient to tilt her head back and open her mouth as wide as possible.

7. With your other hand, depress the patient's tongue with a tongue depressor.

8. Ask the patient to say "Ah."

9. Insert the swab and quickly swab the area of the tonsils.

10. Remove the swab and then the tongue depressor from the patient's mouth.

11. Discard the tongue depressor in the biohazard container.

12. Immediately insert the swab into the plastic sleeve or inoculate the culture plate as required by the test.

13. Crush the vial of transport media or discard after inoculating the culture plate.

14. Label the specimen and arrange for transport to the laboratory or place the plate in the incubator.

15. Remove the gloves and wash your hands.

16. Document the procedure in the patient's chart.

Quick Strep A Test

CRITICAL PROCEDURE STEPS

1. Review the laboratory requisition form and gather the supplies.

2. Confirm the patient's identity and explain the procedure.

3. Wash your hands and don gloves, goggles, and a mask or face shield.
4. Open the testing kit and check the expiration date.
5. Obtain a throat specimen.
6. Complete the quality control tests provided with the testing kit.
7. Put the required amount of the first reagent in the test tube or testing device.
8. Place the swab in the test tube or testing device. Swirl the swab and press it against the sides of the tube or device.
9. Add the second reagent as directed.
10. Read the results at the required time.
11. Appropriately dispose of testing supplies according to OSHA requirements.
12. Remove the gloves and wash your hands.
13. Document the results in the patient's chart.

Specimen Collection Guidelines

YOU SHOULD KNOW

- Obtain the specimen with great care to avoid causing the patient harm, discomfort, or undue embarrassment.
- Collect the material from a site where the organism is most likely to be found and where contamination is least likely to occur.
- Obtain the specimen at a time that allows optimal chance of recovery of the microorganism.

continued

- Use appropriate collection devices, specimen containers, transport systems, and culture media to ensure optimal recovery of microorganisms.
- Obtain a sufficient quantity of the specimen for performing the requested procedures.
- Obtain the specimen before antimicrobial therapy begins.

Transporting to an Outside Laboratory

CRITICAL PROCEDURE STEPS

1. Wash your hands and put on gloves.
2. Obtain the microbiologic culture specimen.
3. Use the collection system specified by the outside laboratory.
4. Label the collection device at the time of collection.
5. Collect the specimen according to the guidelines provided by the laboratory and office policy.
6. Remove the gloves and wash your hands.
7. Complete the requisition form.
8. Place the specimen container in a secondary container or zipper-type plastic bag.
9. Attach the test requisition form to the outside of the secondary container or bag.
10. Log the specimen in the list of outgoing specimens.
11. Store the specimen according to the laboratory guidelines for the type of specimen.
12. Call the laboratory for pickup.
13. At the time of pickup, ensure that all specimens that are logged in are picked up.
14. If you are unsure of collection or transport details, call the laboratory.

SDS

The following information about chemicals can be found on a standard SDS:

- Substance name
- Chemical name
- Common name
- Chemical characteristics
- Physical hazards
- Health hazards
- Guidelines for safe handling
- Emergency and first-aid procedures

Normal Values*

Blood Tests

Blood Test	Normal Range
Blood Counts	
Red blood cells	
Men	$4.7–6.1 \times 10^6$ cells/mcL
Women	$4.2–5.4 \times 10^6$ cells/mcL
White blood cells	$4.5–11.0 \times 10^3$ cells/mcL
Platelets	$150–400 \times 10^3$ cells/mcL
Differential	
Neutrophils	40%–60%
Eosinophils	1%–4%
Basophils	0.5%–1%
Lymphocytes	20%–40%
Monocytes	2%–8%

*Different laboratories may have different normal reference ranges than those represented in this table. Consult your laboratory procedures manual for additional information regarding normal ranges.

Blood Test	Normal Range
Hematocrit	
Men	40.7%–50.3%
Women	36.1%–44.3%
Hemoglobin	
Men	13.8–17.2 g/dL
Women	12.1–15.1 g/dL
Erythrocyte sedimentation rate	
Wintrobe	
Men	0–5 mm/hour
Women	0–15 mm/hour
Westergren	
Men	0–15 mm/hour
Women	0–20 mm/hour
Coagulation tests	
Prothrombin time	11–15 seconds
Bleeding time	2–7 minutes
Electrolytes	
Bicarbonate	27–29 mEq/L (venous plasma)
Calcium	8.6–10.0 mEq/L
Chloride	98–108 mEq/L
Potassium	3.5–5.1 mEq/L
Sodium	136–145 mEq/L
Chemical and Serologic	
Alpha-fetoprotein	
Fetal, first trimester	20–400 mg/dL
Adult	<15 ng/mL

Blood Test	Normal Range
Alanine aminotransferase	
Men	10–40 U/L
Women	7–35 U/L
Aspartate aminotransferase	
Men	11–26 U/L
Women	10–20 U/L
Bilirubin	0.3–1.2 mg/dL
Blood urea nitrogen (BUN)	6–20 mg/dL
Carcinoembryonic antigen	<5.0 ng/mL
Cholesterol, total	
Men	158–277 mg/dL
Women	162–285 mg/dL
HDL	
Men	28–63 mg/dL
Women	37–92 mg/dL
LDL	
Men	89–197 mg/dL
Women	88–201 mg/dL
Creatine kinase	
Men	38–174 U/L
Women	26–140 U/L
Creatinine	
Men	0.9–1.3 mg/dL
Women	0.6–1.2 mg/dL
Cytomegalovirus	None

continued

Blood Test	Normal Range
Epstein-Barr virus	None
Fibrinogen	200–400 mg/dL
Glucose (FBS)	74–120 mg/dL
Group A strep	None
HIV	None
Insulin	<17 mcU/mL

Iron, total
  Men
  Women
	
	65–175 mcg/dL
	50–170 mcg/dL

Lactate dehydrogenase	140–280 U/L
pH	7.32–7.43 (venous blood)

Proteins
  Total
  Albumin
	
	6.2–8.0 g/dL
	3.4–4.8 g/dL

Uric acid
  Men
  Women
	
	4.4–7.6 mg/dL
	2.3–6.6 mg/dL

Urinalysis

Physical Characteristics	
Test	Normal Values
Color	Pale yellow–yellow
Clarity	Clear–slightly turbid

Reagent Strip Test*	
Test	**Normal Values**
Bilirubin	Negative
Blood	Negative
Glucose	Negative
Ketone bodies (acetone)	Negative
Leukocytes	Negative
Nitrites	Negative
pH	4.5–8.0
Protein	Negative–trace
Specific gravity	1.002–1.028
Urobilinogen	0.3–1.0 EU
Microscopic Examination	
Test	**Normal Value**
Bacteria	Negative
Casts	
Epithelial cell	Negative
Granular	Negative
Hyaline	Few
Red blood cell	Negative
Waxy	Negative
White blood cell	Negative

*Individual laboratories may use different reference values or reagent strips. Consult the reference values provided by the lab or the manufacturer of the reagent strips.

continued

Microscopic Examination	
Test	**Normal Value**
Crystals	
Amorphous phosphates	Normal
Calcium carbonate	Normal
Calcium oxalate	Normal
Cholesterol	Negative
Cystine	Negative
Leucine	Negative
Sulfonamide	Negative
Triple phosphate	Normal
Tyrosine	Negative
Uric acid	Normal
Epithelial cells	
Renal	Negative
Squamous, adult females	Moderate
Squamous, adult males	Few
Transitional	Rare
Mucus	Rare–few
Protozoa	Negative
Red blood cells	0–3/high-power field
White blood cells	0–8/high-power field
Yeast	Few

24-Hour	
Test	Normal Value
5HIAA	2–8 mg
Albumin (quantitative)	10–140 mg/L
Ammonia	140–1,500 mg
Calcium (quantitative)	100–300 mg
Catecholamines, total	<100 mcg
Chloride	110–120 mEq
Cortisol	10 to 100 mcg
Creatine, nonpregnant women/men	<100 mcg
Creatine, pregnant women	≤12% of creatinine
Creatinine, men	1.0–1.9 g
Creatinine, women	0.8–1.7 g
Cystine and cysteine	<38.1 mg
Glucose (quantitative)	50–500 mg
Phosphorus	0.4–1.3 g
Potassium	25–120 mEq/L
Protein (Bence-Jones)	Negative
Sodium	80–180 mEq

continued

24-Hour	
Test	Normal Value
Urea nitrogen	6–17 g
Uric acid	0.25–0.75 g
Urobilinogen (quantitative)	1.0–4.0 mg
Volume, adult females	600–1,600 mL
Volume, adult males	800–1,800 mL
Volume, children	3–4 times adult rate/kg

Safety

Accident Reporting Guidelines for Reporting Blood and Body Fluid Exposure

1. Immediate cleaning of the area, including disinfection of contaminated surfaces and sterilization of contaminated instruments and equipment
2. Notification of a designated emergency contact, as identified in your office's safety manual
3. Documentation of the incident on a form, including the names of all parties involved, the names of witnesses, a description of the incident, and a record of medical treatments given to those involved
4. Medical evaluation and follow-up exam of the employees involved
5. Written evaluation of the medical condition of the involved individuals as well as testing for infection, provided that such testing does not violate confidentiality regulations

Biologic Safety

- Follow standard precautions.
- If you have cuts, lesions, or sores, do not expose yourself to potentially contaminated material.
- Wash your hands before and after every procedure.
- Wear gloves at all times. Wear other protective gear as appropriate.
- Always use an approved pipette device to transfer fluids. Never pipette by mouth.
- Work in a biologic safety cabinet when splashes or sprays are possible.
- When transferring a blood sample from one container to another, take care when opening the tube. Open the tube away from your face.
- Establish clean and dirty areas in the laboratory.
- Disinfect the work area with 10% bleach at least once a day.
- Dispose of waste materials immediately.
- Dispose of sharps in approved containers.
- Decontaminate equipment prior to servicing.
- If you use a bleach solution for disinfection, change it daily.

Chemical Safety

- Wear protective gear.
- Carry chemical containers with both hands.
- Work in a properly ventilated area.
- If you must smell a chemical, hold it away from your nose and fan air across the container toward your nose.
- Work inside a fume hood if the chemical vapor is hazardous.

- Wear a personal ventilation device when indicated by the SDS.
- Never combine chemicals in ways not specifically required in test procedures.
- Always use an approved pipette device to transfer fluids. Never pipette by mouth.
- If you are combining acid with other substances, always add acid to the other substance.
- Clean up spills according to strict hazardous waste control procedures.
- Never touch an unknown chemical substance with your bare hands.

Electrical Safety

- Avoid using extension cords.
- Repair or replace equipment that has a broken or frayed cord.
- Dry your hands before working with electrical devices.
- Do not position electrical devices near sinks, faucets, or other sources of water.

Fire Safety

- Extinguish an open flame immediately after use.
- Keep hair, clothing, and jewelry away from an open flame.
- When using a chemical near an open flame, check the SDS to identify the level of risk of fire for that chemical.
- Never lean over an open flame.
- Never leave an open flame unattended.
- Turn off gas valves immediately after use.

Handling a Fire Emergency

CRITICAL PROCEDURE STEPS

1. In the case of a fire, pull the fire alarm or call emergency services.
2. Move patients out of the area.
3. Remove the fire extinguisher from its stored location.
4. Assess the fire.

If the Fire Cannot Be Easily Contained

5. Calmly and quickly ask each employee to follow the established fire plan.
6. Remove all patients to the outside of the building, ensuring patient comfort and safety.

If the Fire Is Small and Easily Contained

7. Hold the fire extinguisher upright.
8. **P**ull the safety pin on the fire extinguisher.
9. **A**im at the base of the fire.
10. **S**queeze the trigger.
11. **S**weep from side to side until the fire is out.
12. Do not reenter the area until the fire department assesses and clears the area.

Needlestick Prevention

- Healthcare employers must evaluate new safety-engineered control devices on an annual basis and implement the use of devices that reasonably reduce the risk of needlestick injuries.

- Healthcare facilities must maintain a detailed log of sharps injuries that are incurred from contaminated sharps.
- Healthcare employers must solicit input from employees involved in direct patient care to identify, evaluate, and implement engineering and work practice controls.

Safe Injection Practices

- Use aseptic technique to avoid contamination of sterile injection equipment.
- Clean the top of medication vials with 70% isopropyl alcohol before withdrawing medications.
- Do not administer medications from a syringe to multiple patients.
- Use single-dose vials for parenteral medications whenever possible.
- Do not administer medications from single-dose vials or ampules to multiple patients or combine leftover contents for later use.
- If multi-dose vials must be used, both the needle or cannula and syringe used to access the multi-dose vial must be sterile.
- Do not keep multi-dose vials in the immediate patient treatment area and store in accordance with the manufacturer's recommendations; discard if sterility is compromised or questionable.

Physical Safety

- Walk, do not run, in the laboratory.
- Close all cabinet and closet doors and all desk and worktable drawers.
- Never use damaged equipment or supplies.
- Do not overextend your reach when attempting to grasp supplies.

- Do not climb onto chairs, desks, or tables to reach anything.
- Lift with your legs when lifting heavy objects.
- Adjust your seat to the correct position to avoid back strain.
- Do not eat or drink in the laboratory.
- Do not put anything in your mouth while working in the laboratory.
- Do not apply makeup or lip balm or insert contact lenses in the laboratory.
- Know the location of the first-aid kit.
- Know the location and proper use of the eyewash and shower stations.

Maintaining and Using an Eyewash Station

On a weekly basis:

1. Check that the path to the eyewash station is clear and no more than 10 seconds from the hazard.
2. Ensure that the "Eyewash" sign is easily visible.
3. Make sure the covers are in place.
4. Ensure that the unit comes on within 1 second and stays on once it is activated.
5. Check the flow of the eyewash to ensure that it has sufficient flow to wash the eye but is not so strong it will damage the eye tissues.
6. Check that the temperature of the water is above 60°F and below 100°F.
7. Flush the system for 1 minute.
8. Complete the safety inspection record attached to the eyewash station.

During a splash or splatter emergency:

1. Help the victim to the eyewash station.
2. Activate the system.
3. If the eyewash is a plumbed unit, have the victim lean into the eyewash, keeping her eyes continuously open. Don gloves and gown and assist the victim as needed.
4. Continuously flush the eyes for at least 15 minutes or the length of time recommended on the SDS, if applicable.
5. Alert the physician or EMS.

Slide Staining Techniques

Gram Stain

CRITICAL PROCEDURE STEPS

1. Assemble all necessary supplies.
2. Wash your hands and don gloves.
3. Place the heat-fixed smear on a level staining rack and tray, smear side up.
4. Completely cover the specimen area with crystal violet stain.
5. Allow the stain to sit for 1 minute; then rinse with distilled water.
6. Using forceps, tilt the slide to one side to drain the excess water.
7. Place the slide flat on the rack again and cover with iodine solution.

8. Allow the iodine to sit for 1 minute; then rinse with distilled water.

9. Using forceps, tilt the slide to drain the excess water.

10. With the slide tilted, apply the alcohol drop by drop until no more purple washes off (10–30 seconds).

11. Rinse the slide with distilled water; then tilt it to remove excess water.

12. Return the slide to the rack and cover with safranin stain.

13. Allow the safranin to sit for 1 minute; then rinse with distilled water.

14. Carefully wipe the back of the slide to remove excess stain.

15. Place the slide in the vertical position and allow to air-dry or blot lightly with blotting paper.

16. Sanitize and disinfect the work area.

17. Remove the gloves and wash your hands.

Troubleshooting Lab Procedures

General Steps

- Have a written procedure for troubleshooting tests and equipment.
- Recognize the problem (controls give clues to possible problems).
- Think about possible causes.
- Start with the simplest cause first.

- Document your findings.
- Call your service company after you have checked everything you know to check.

Laboratory Equipment

- Check the power source at the machine, the wall outlet, the breaker box, or the battery.
- Check the equipment manual for troubleshooting information.
- Reboot the equipment by turning it off, waiting a few minutes, and then turning it back on.
- Check the service log for the date of the last maintenance.
- If you are able to repair the problem, run controls to verify that the problem is fixed before testing patient samples.

Laboratory Test Kits

- Read the package insert to verify that you have performed the test correctly.
- Check to make sure that you have used the correct reagents or test strips.
- Check the dates on the reagents or test strips to make sure that they are not outdated.
- Make sure that you are using the proper sample for the test.
- Repeat the test using control samples.
- If the controls are correct, repeat the test with the patient sample.

Stool Specimens

Fecal Occult Blood Testing

CRITICAL PROCEDURE STEPS

1. Confirm the patient's identity and ensure that all forms are completed correctly.
2. Label the occult blood testing card or slide. Give the patient the test card or slide and collecting spoon or applicator.
3. Give the patient pretest and collection instructions.

Processing the Test

4. Wash your hands and don gloves.
5. Open the back of the card. Add the recommended amount of developing reagent directly over the smeared area on the back side of the paper and over the positive and negative controls, if present on the card.
6. Read the test results at the appropriate time.
7. Dispose of the testing card according to OSHA regulations.
8. Remove the gloves and wash your hands.
9. Document the results in the patient's chart.

Urine

Characteristics

- **Color and turbidity**—assess for color and cloudiness
- **Odor**—should be aromatic but not unpleasant

- **Specific gravity**—a measure of the concentration or amount of substances dissolved in urine
- **Volume**—usually measured on a timed specimen

Collecting a Clean Catch Mid-Stream Urine Specimen

CRITICAL PROCEDURE STEPS

1. Confirm the patient's identity and be sure that all forms are correctly completed.
2. Label the sterile urine specimen container with the patient's name, ID number, and date of birth; the licensed practitioner's name; the date and time of collection; and the initials of the person collecting the specimen.

When the patient will be completing the procedure independently:

3. Explain the procedure in detail. Provide the patient with written instructions, antiseptic towelettes, and the labeled sterile specimen container.
4. Confirm that the patient understands the instructions, especially not to touch the inside of the specimen container and to refrigerate the specimen until it is brought to the licensed practitioner's office.

When you are assisting a patient:

3. Explain the procedure and how you will be assisting in the collection.
4. Wash your hands and put on exam gloves.

When you are assisting in the collection for female patients:

5. Remove the lid from the specimen container and place the lid upside-down on a flat surface.

6. Use three antiseptic towelettes to clean the perineal area by spreading the labia and wiping from front to back. Wipe with the first towelette on one side and discard it. Wipe with the second towelette on the other side and discard it. Wipe with the third towelette down the middle and discard it. To remove soap residue that could cause a higher pH and affect chemical test results, rinse the area once from front to back with water.

7. Keeping the patient's labia spread to avoid contamination, tell her to urinate into the toilet. After she has expressed a small amount of urine, instruct her to stop the flow.

8. Position the specimen container close to but not touching the patient.

9. Tell the patient to start urinating again. Collect the necessary amount of urine in the container. (If the patient cannot stop her urine flow, move the container into the urine flow and collect the specimen anyway.)

10. Allow the patient to finish urinating. Place the lid back on the collection container.

11. Remove the gloves and wash your hands.

12. Complete the test requisition slip and record the collection in the patient's chart.

When you are assisting in the collection for male patients:

5. Remove the lid from the specimen container and place the lid upside-down on a flat surface.

continued

6. If the patient is circumcised, use an antiseptic towelette to clean the head of the penis. Wipe with a second towelette directly across the urethral opening. If the patient is uncircumcised, retract the foreskin before cleaning the penis. To remove soap residue that could cause a higher pH and affect chemical test results, rinse the area once from front to back with water.

7. Keeping an uncircumcised patient's foreskin retracted, tell the patient to urinate into the toilet. After he has expressed a small amount of urine, instruct him to stop the flow.

8. Position the specimen container close to but not touching the patient.

9. Tell the patient to start urinating again. Collect the necessary amount of urine in the container. (If the patient cannot stop his urine flow, move the container into the urine flow and collect the specimen anyway.)

10. Allow the patient to finish urinating. Place the lid back on the collection container.

11. Remove the gloves and wash your hands.

12. Complete the laboratory requisition form and record the collection in the patient's chart/progress note.

Collecting a Urine Specimen from a Pediatric Patient

CRITICAL PROCEDURE STEPS

1. Confirm the patient's identity and be sure all forms are correctly completed.
2. Explain the procedure to the child (if age-appropriate) and to the parents or guardians.
3. Wash your hands and put on exam gloves.
4. Have the parents pull the child's pants down and take off the diaper.
5. Position the child with the genitalia exposed.
6. Clean the genitalia. For a male patient, wipe the tip of the penis with a soapy cotton ball, and then rinse it with a cotton ball saturated with sterile water. Allow to air-dry. For a female patient, use soapy cotton balls to clean the labia majora from front to back, using one cotton ball for each wipe. Again, use cotton balls saturated in sterile water to rinse the area, and allow it to air-dry.
7. Remove the paper backing from the plastic urine collection bag and apply the sticky, adhesive surface over the penis and scrotum (in a male patient) or vulva (in a female patient). Seal tightly to avoid leaks. Do not include the child's rectum within the collection bag or cover it with the adhesive surface.
8. Diaper the child.
9. Remove the gloves and wash your hands.
10. Check the collection bag every half-hour for urine. You must open the diaper to check; do not just feel the diaper.

continued

11. If the child has voided, wash your hands and put on exam gloves.

12. Remove the diaper, take off the urine collection bag very carefully so that you do not irritate the child's skin, wash off the adhesive residue, rinse, and pat dry.

13. Diaper the child.

14. Place the specimen in the specimen container and cover it.

15. Label the urine specimen container with the patient's name, ID number, and date of birth; the physician's name; the date and time of collection; and your initials.

16. Remove the gloves and wash your hands.

17. Complete the laboratory requisition form, and record the collection in the patient's chart.

YOU SHOULD KNOW

24-Hour Urine Specimen Patient Instructions

- At the start of the observation period (usually early in the morning), void and discard the first urine specimen. This will start the collection period. Write the start date and time on the urine specimen storage containers.

- Do not discard the preservative in the urine specimen storage container.

- For the next 24 hours, each time you void, collect the entire specimen in the provided specimen collection container.

- Carefully transfer the entire specimen in the urine storage container, being careful not to spill any urine. If you spill urine or accidently urinate in the toilet, call to reschedule the test.
- Keep the specimen covered and in the refrigerator or in a cooler when not in use.
- Twenty-four hours after you begin the test, void once more and transfer to the specimen storage container. Write the end date and time on the container.
- As quickly as possible, bring the specimen back to the office or deliver it to the laboratory if instructed to do so. Keep the specimen cool during transport.

Color and Turbidity: Possible Causes

Color and Turbidity	Possible Causes
Colorless or pale	Diabetes, anxiety, chronic renal disease, diuretic therapy, excessive fluid intake
Cloudy	Infection, inflammation, glomerular nephritis, vegetarian diet
Milky white	Fats, pus, amorphous phosphates, spermatozoa
Dark yellow, dark amber	Acute febrile disease, vomiting or diarrhea, low fluid intake, excessive sweating
Yellow-brown	Excessive RBC destruction, bile duct obstruction, diminished liver cell function, bilirubin

continued

Color and Turbidity	Possible Causes
Orange-yellow, orange-red, orange-brown	Excessive RBC destruction, diminished liver cell function, bile, hepatitis, urobilinuria, obstructive jaundice, hematuria
Salmon pink	Amorphous urates
Cloudy red	RBCs, excessive destruction of skeletal or cardiac muscle
Bright yellow or red	RBCs, excessive destruction of skeletal or cardiac muscle, porphyria, beets, some drugs, dyes
Dark red, red-brown	Porphyria, RBCs, blood from previous hemorrhage
Green, blue-green	Biliverdin, *Pseudomonas* organisms, oxidation of bilirubin
Green-brown	Bile duct obstruction
Brownish black	Methemoglobin, melanin, some drugs
Dark brown or black	Acute glomerulonephritis, some drugs

Reagent Strip Testing Method

CRITICAL PROCEDURE STEPS

1. Wash your hands and put on gloves.
2. Check the specimen for proper labeling and visible contaminants.
3. Check the expiration date on the strips.
4. Check the strip for damage.

5. Complete the test within 1 hour of collecting the sample, or refrigerate the sample until the test can be performed.
6. Swirl the sample.
7. Dip the strip in the urine, completely covering the strip.
8. Tap the strip sideways on a paper towel but do not blot it.
9. Read the strip against the chart at the designated time.
10. Record the values on the laboratory report form.
11. Discard the used disposable supplies.
12. Clean and disinfect the work area.
13. Remove your gloves and wash your hands.
14. Record the results in the patient's chart/progress note.

Establishing a Chain of Custody

CRITICAL PROCEDURE STEPS

1. Positively identify the patient. (Complete the top part of the chain-of-custody form with the name and address of the drug-testing laboratory, the name and address of the requesting company, and the Social Security number of the patient. Make a note on the form if the patient refuses to give her Social Security number.) Ensure that the number on the printed label matches the number at the top of the form.
2. Ensure that the patient removes any outer clothing and empties her pockets, displaying all items.

continued

3. Instruct the patient to wash and dry her hands.

4. Instruct the patient that no water is to be running while the specimen is being collected. Tape the faucet handles in the off position and add bluing agent to the toilet.

5. Instruct the patient to provide the specimen as soon as it is collected so that you can record the temperature of the specimen.

6. Remain by the door of the restroom.

7. Measure and record the temperature of the urine specimen within 4 minutes of collection. Make a note if its temperature is out of acceptable range.

8. Examine the specimen for signs of adulteration (unusual color or odor).

9. *In the presence of the patient,* check the "single specimen" or "split specimen" box. The patient should witness your transferring the specimen into the transport specimen bottle(s), capping the bottle(s), and affixing the label on the bottle(s).

10. The patient should initial the specimen bottle label(s) *after* it is placed on the bottle(s).

11. Complete any additional information requested on the form, including the authorization for drug screening, including the following:
    - Patient's daytime telephone number
    - Patient's evening telephone number
    - Test requested
    - Patient's name
    - Patient's signature
    - Date

12. Sign the CCF; print your full name and, note the date and time of the collection and the name of the courier service.
13. Give the patient a copy of the CCF.
14. Place the specimen in a leakproof bag with the appropriate copy of the form.
15. Release the specimen to the courier service.
16. Distribute additional copies as required.

Microscopic Components

The microscopic components of urine include the following:

- Bacteria
- Casts
- Cells
- Crystals
- Parasites
- Yeasts

Centrifuging to Obtain Urine Sediment

CRITICAL PROCEDURE STEPS

1. Wash your hands and put on gloves.
2. Check the specimen for proper labeling and visible contaminants.
3. Complete the test within 1 hour of collecting the sample, or refrigerate the sample until the test can be performed.

continued

4. Swirl the sample.
5. Pour 10 mL of the urine in one test tube.
6. Place the tube in the centrifuge and balance with another tube filled with 10 mL of water.
7. Secure the centrifuge lid and set the timer.
8. Set the speed according to office protocol and start the centrifuge.
9. After the centrifuge stops, lift the tube and carefully pour off the liquid.
10. Tap to resuspend the sediment in the drops of urine left in the bottom of the tube.
11. Use a pipette to remove a few drops of the urine sediment.
12. Place the drops on a clean slide and cover with a coverslip.
13. Place the slide on the microscope stage and focus the image.
14. Alert the physician that the slide has been prepared and is ready for examination.

Anatomy and Physiology

Anatomical Position

- The body is standing upright and facing forward with the arms at the sides and the palms of the hands and toes facing forward.
- This position is used as a reference point when describing directional terms.

Body Cavities

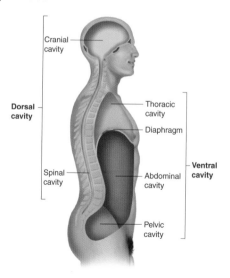

Body Movements

Flexion—bending a body part or decreasing the angle of a joint

Extension—straightening a body part or increasing the angle of a joint

Hyperextension—extending a body part past the normal anatomical position

Dorsiflexion—pointing the toes up

Plantar flexion—pointing the toes down

Abduction—moving a body part away from the midline of the body

Adduction—moving a body part toward the midline of the body

Rotation—twisting a body part; for example, turning your head from side to side

Circumduction—moving a body part in a circle; for example, moving your arm in a circular motion

Pronation—turning the palm of the hand down or lying face down

Supination—turning the palm of the hand up or lying face up

Inversion—turning the sole of the foot medially

Eversion—turning the sole of the foot laterally

Protraction—moving a body part anteriorly

Retraction—moving a body part posteriorly

Depression—lowering a body part; for example, lowering your shoulders

Elevation—lifting a body part; for example, elevating your shoulders as in a shrugging expression

Body Planes

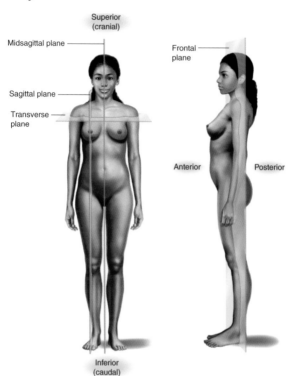

Body Quadrants and Regions

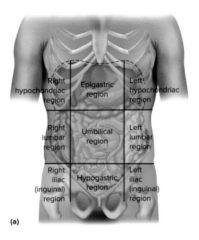

(a)

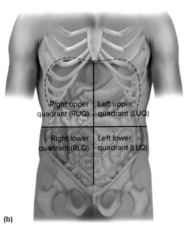

(b)

Directional Terms

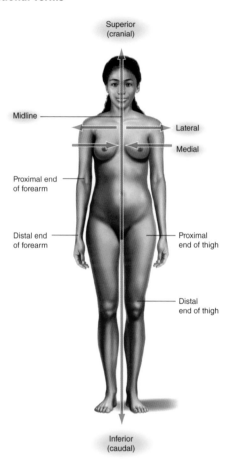

Superior (cranial)

Midline

Lateral

Medial

Proximal end of forearm

Distal end of forearm

Proximal end of thigh

Distal end of thigh

Inferior (caudal)

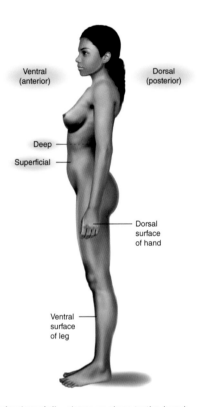

Ventral
(anterior)

Dorsal
(posterior)

Deep

Superficial

Dorsal
surface
of hand

Ventral
surface
of leg

Superior (cranial)—above or close to the head

Inferior (caudal)—below or close to the feet

Anterior (ventral)—toward the front of the body

Posterior (dorsal)—toward the back of the body

Medial—closer to the midline of the body

Lateral—farther away from the midline of the body

Proximal—closer to a point of attachment or to the trunk of the body

Distal—farther away from a point of attachment or from the trunk of the body

Superficial—close to the surface of the body

Deep—more internal

Organization of the Body

Atoms—the simplest units of all matter

Matter—anything that takes up space and has weight; includes liquids, solids, and gases

Molecule—the smallest unit into which an element can be divided and still retain its properties; it is formed when atoms bond together

Organelle—a structure within a cell that performs a specific function

Cell—the smallest living units of structure and function

Tissue—a structure that is formed when similar types of cells organize together

Organ—a structure formed by the organization of two or more different tissue types that carries out specific functions

Organ system—a system that consists of organs that join together to carry out vital functions

Organism—a whole living being that is formed from organ systems

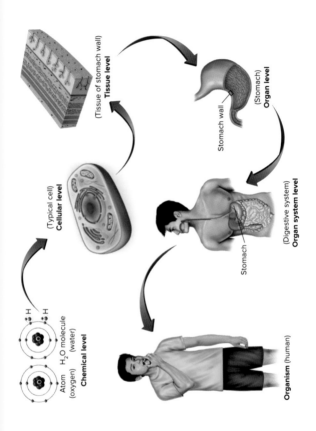

Chemical level
Atom (oxygen)
H₂O molecule (water)

Cellular level
(Typical cell)

Tissue level
(Tissue of stomach wall)

Organ level
(Stomach)
Stomach wall

Organ system level
(Digestive system)
Stomach

Organism (human)

240

Organ Systems

The integumentary system

- Functions—protection, body temperature regulation, vitamin D precursor production, sensation, and prevention of water loss
- Organs—skin, hair, sebaceous glands, nails, and sudoriferous glands

The skeletal system

- Functions—shape, support, protection, movement, blood cell production, and storage of minerals and fat
- Organs—bones, associated cartilages, ligaments, and joints

The muscular system

- Functions—movement, stability and posture, control of body openings, and heat production
- Organs—muscles and tendons

The cardiovascular system

- Functions—transport of blood, nutrients, waste products, and hormones; immune response; regulation of body temperature
- Organs—heart, blood, veins, arteries, venules, arterioles, and capillaries

The respiratory system

- Functions—oxygen and carbon dioxide exchange, regulation of blood pH
- Organs—nose, pharynx, larynx, trachea, bronchial tree, and lungs

The nervous system
- Functions—detecting sensations and controlling movements, physiologic processes, and intellectual functions
- Organs—brain, spinal cord, nerves, and sensory receptors

The urinary system
- Functions—removal of waste products from the blood, urine elimination, regulation of blood cell production and blood pH, blood pressure regulation, and ion and water balance
- Organs—kidneys, ureters, bladder, and urethra

The reproductive systems
- Function—offspring production
- Organs
  - Male—testes, penis, prostate gland, bulbourethral glands accessory structures, and ducts
  - Female—ovaries, fallopian tubes, uterus, vagina, mammary glands, and associated structures

The lymphatic and immune systems
- Function—protect the body against infections, toxins, and cancer
- Organs—spleen, thymus, lymph nodes, lymphatic vessels, and lymph

The digestive system
- Functions—digestion and absorption of nutrients and waste elimination
- Organs—mouth, teeth, salivary glands, pharynx, esophagus, stomach, small intestine, large intestine, pancreas, liver, and gallbladder

The endocrine system

- Function—regulation of all cellular chemical reactions
- Organs—glands that secrete hormones, such as hypothalamus, pituitary, pineal body, thyroid, parathyroid, thymus, adrenals, and pancreas

Communication

5 Cs of Communication

- **Completeness**—the message must contain all necessary information.
- **Clarity**—the message must be legible and free from ambiguity.
- **Conciseness**—the message must be brief and direct.
- **Courtesy**—the message must be respectful and considerate of others.
- **Cohesiveness**—the message must be organized and logical.

Telephone Screening and Procedures

Calls requiring the licensed practitioner's attention

- Emergency calls
- Calls from other providers
- Patient requests to discuss test results, particularly abnormal results
- Reports from patients concerning unsatisfactory progress
- Requests for prescription renewals (unless previously authorized on the patient's chart)
- Personal calls

Collecting patient data

Effective methods of collecting patient data include the following:

- Asking open-ended questions
- Asking hypothetical questions
- Mirroring a patient's responses and verbalizing the implied
- Focusing on the patient
- Encouraging the patient to take the lead
- Encouraging the patient to provide additional information
- Encouraging the patient to evaluate his situation

Documenting a phone call

Each call should have the following information documented:

- Date and time of the call
- Name of the person for whom you took the message
- Caller's name
- Caller's telephone number (including area code and extension, if any)
- Description or action to be taken, including comments such as "Urgent," "Please call back," "Wants to see you," "Will call back," or "Returned your call"
- The complete message
- Name or initials of the person taking the call

Handling incoming calls

- Answer the telephone promptly by the third ring. Hold the telephone to your ear or use a headset to hold the earpiece securely against your ear. Do not cradle the telephone with your shoulder; doing so can cause muscle strain.

- Hold the mouthpiece about an inch away from your mouth, and leave one hand free to write with.
- Greet the caller first with the name of the medical office and then with your name.
- Identify the caller. Demonstrate your willingness to assist the caller by asking, "How may I help you?"
- Be courteous, calm, and pleasant, no matter how hurried you are.
- Identify the nature of the call and devote your full attention to the caller.
- At the end of the call, say goodbye and use the caller's name. Let the caller hang up first.

Handling outgoing calls

- Plan before you call. Have all the information you need in front of you before you dial the telephone number. Plan what you will say and decide what questions to ask so that you will not have to call back for additional information.
- Double-check the telephone number. If you dial a wrong number, apologize for the mistake.
- Allow enough time, at least a minute or about eight rings, for someone to answer the telephone. When calling patients who are elderly or physically disabled, allow additional time.
- Identify yourself. Give your name and state that you are calling on behalf of the licensed practitioner or the practice.
- Ask if you have called at a convenient time and whether the person has time to talk with you. If it is not a good time, ask when you should call back.
- Be ready to speak as soon as the person you called answers the telephone. Do not waste the person's time while you collect your thoughts.

- If you are calling to give information, ask if the person has a pencil and piece of paper available. Do not begin with dates, times, or instructions until the person is ready to write down the information.

Telephone Etiquette

Checking for understanding
- If a call is long or complicated, summarize what was said to be sure that both you and the caller understand the information.
- Ask if the caller has any questions about what you have discussed.

Communicating feelings
- When dealing with a caller who is nervous, upset, or angry, try to show empathy.
- Communicating with empathy helps the caller feel more positive about the conversation and the medical office.

Enunciation
- Speak clearly and distinctly.
- Do not chew gum or eat while on the phone.
- Do not prop the phone between your ear and shoulder.

Exhibiting courtesy
- Project an attitude of helpfulness.
- Always use the person's name during the conversation.
- Apologize for any errors or delays.
- When ending the conversation, be sure to thank the caller before hanging up.

Giving undivided attention
- Do not try to answer the telephone while continuing to carry out another task.

- Give the caller the same undivided attention you would if the person were in the office.
- Listen carefully to get the correct information.

Handling difficult situations
- If an emergency arises while you are on the phone, ask if you can call back.
- Explain that you are currently handling an urgent matter.
- Offer to return the call in a few minutes.

Making a good impression
- How you handle telephone calls will have an impact on the public image of the medical practice.

Putting a call on hold
- Before putting a call on hold, always let the caller state the reason for the call.
- State why you need to place the call on hold.
- Explain how long you expect the wait to be.
- Ask the caller if this wait is acceptable.
- If you need to answer a second call, get the second caller's name and telephone number, and put that call on hold until you have completed the first call.

Pronunciation
- Say the words correctly.
- You may have to ask a patient to pronounce his or her name.

Remembering patients' names
- When patients are recognized by name, they are more likely to have positive feelings about the practice.
- Using a caller's name during a conversation makes the caller feel important.

Tone

- Speak with a positive and respectful tone.

Your telephone voice

- Speak directly into the receiver; otherwise, your voice will be difficult to understand.
- Smile. The smile in your voice will convey your friendliness and willingness to help.
- Visualize the caller, and speak directly to that person.
- Convey a friendly and respectful interest in the caller.
- You should sound helpful and alert.
- Use language that is nontechnical and easy to understand. Never use slang.
- Speak at a natural pace, not too quickly or too slowly.
- Use a normal conversational tone.
- Vary your pitch while you are talking.
- Make the caller feel important.

Ending the conversation

- Take a few seconds to complete the call so that the caller feels properly cared for and satisfied.
- Complete the call by summarizing the important points of the conversation and thanking the caller.
- Let the caller hang up first.

Telephone Triage

Definition: A process for deciding what necessary action to take

Tips for Taking Messages

- Always have a pen or pencil and paper on hand.
- Jot down notes as the information is given.

- Verify information, especially the spelling of patient or caller names and the correct spelling of medications.
- Verify the correct callback number.
- When taking a phone message, never make a commitment on behalf of the intended recipient by saying, "I'll have him call you." An appropriate response would be "I will give your message to Dr. Buckwalter."

Ergonomics/Body Mechanics

Body Mechanics Rules

- Lift with your strongest muscles, including your legs and arms, rather than your back.
- Keep your feet apart when lifting and moving.
- Bend from the hips and knees.

Patient Transfer from a Wheelchair

CRITICAL PROCEDURE STEPS

Never risk injuring yourself; call for assistance when in doubt. As a rule, you should not attempt to lift more than 35% of your body weight.

Preparation Before Transfer

1. Identify the patient and introduce yourself.
2. Wash your hands.
3. Explain the procedure in detail.
4. Position the wheelchair at a right angle to the end of the examining table. This position reduces the distance between the wheelchair and the end of the examining table across which the patient must move.

continued

5. Lock the wheels of the wheelchair to prevent the wheelchair from moving during the transfer.

6. Lift the patient's feet and fold back the foot and leg supports of the wheelchair.

7. Place the patient's feet on the floor, and ensure that the patient will not slip on the floor. (The patient should have shoes or slippers with nonskid soles.) Place your feet in front of the patient's feet to prevent further slipping.

8. If needed, place a step-stool in front of the table, and place the patient's feet flat on the stool.

Transferring the Patient by Yourself

9. Face the patient, spread your feet apart, align your knees with the patient's knees, and bend your knees slightly. (If you lift while bending at the waist instead of bending your knees, you can cause serious injury to your back.)

10. Have the patient hold on to your shoulders.

11. Place your arms around the patient, under the patient's arms.

12. Tell the patient that you will lift on the count of three, and ask the patient to support as much of his own weight as possible (if he is able).

13. At the count of three, lift the patient.

14. Pivot the patient to bring the back of the patient's knees against the table.

15. Gently lower the patient into a sitting position on the table. If the patient cannot sit unassisted, help him move into a supine position.

16. Move the wheelchair out of the way.

17. Assist the patient with disrobing as necessary, providing a gown and drape.

Transferring the Patient with Assistance

18. Working with your partner, both of you face the patient, spread your feet apart, position yourselves so that one of each of your knees is aligned with the patient's knees, and bend your knees slightly. (If you lift while bending at your waist instead of bending your knees, you can cause serious injury to your back.)

19. Have the patient place one hand on each of your shoulders and hold on.

20. Each of you places your outermost arm around the patient, one under each of the patient's arms. Then interlock your wrists.

21. Tell the patient that you will lift on the count of three, and ask the patient to support as much of his own weight as possible (if he is able).

22. At the count of three, you should lift the patient together.

23. The stronger of the two of you should pivot the patient to bring the back of the patient's knees against the table.

24. Working together, gently lower the patient into a sitting position on the table. If the patient cannot sit unassisted, help him move into a supine position.

25. Move the wheelchair out of the way.

26. Assist the patient with disrobing as necessary, providing a gown and drape.

Computer Ergonomics

When using a keyboard for extended periods, you should practice proper techniques to prevent carpal tunnel syndrome.

- While seated, hold your arms relaxed at your sides, and check to make sure that your keyboard is positioned slightly higher than your elbows. As you input, keep your elbows at your sides and relax your shoulders.
- Use only your fingers to press keys, and do not use more pressure than necessary. Use a wrist rest, and keep your wrists relaxed and straight.
- To strike difficult-to-reach keys, move your whole hand rather than stretching your fingers. To press two keys at the same time, such as "Control" and "F1," use two hands.
- Break up long periods of keyboard work with other tasks that do not require computer use.

Tips for Relieving Symptoms

If you have symptoms of carpal tunnel syndrome, try these suggestions for relief.

- Elevate your arms.
- Wear a splint on the hand and forearm.
- Discuss your symptoms with a licensed provider, who may prescribe medication.

Electronic Health Records (EHR)

Meaningful Use

Meaningful use is using certified electronic health record (EHR) technology to

- Improve quality, safety, efficiency, and reduce health disparities.
- Engage patients and family.

- Improve care coordination, and population and public health.
- Maintain privacy and security of patient health information.

Advantages of EHR Programs

- **Access**—healthcare providers can access electronic records at various locations, including the laboratory, pharmacy, and even the medical records department.
- **Availability**—information is immediately available, so healthcare providers do not have to wait for paper documents to be written and sent. The data can be viewed at any electronic record location immediately upon entry.
- **Security**—Electronic records provide security because they require passwords for each individual entering the records. Passwords allow each type of healthcare provider access to only the information he or she requires in his or her position.
- **Safety**—sophisticated programs help prevent patient identification errors by including a photograph of each patient as part of the patient record.
- **Extra features**—electronic software programs can alert the healthcare provider to abnormal test results or the need for routine tests to be performed. More sophisticated programs can document health trends, provide voice recognition, and convert notes to complete sentences.

Additional EHR Functions

In addition to housing patient medical records, many EHR programs also function in the following capacities:

- **Reminders**—tickler files remind you of important events or individual patient requirements.
- **Specialty-specific**—EHR programs can be modified to allow individual practices to "mold" the program to the specialty needs of the practice.

- **Electronic schedulers**—schedulers are often included in EHR programs as an added bonus—no more appointment book!
- **Insurance eligibility and verification programs**—these programs allow for online coverage and benefit verification, avoiding the need for staff to wait on hold to speak with a customer service representative to obtain the required information.
- **Billing and coding programs**—billing and coding interfaces "speak" to the medical record so that coding occurs automatically based on the practitioner's medical record documentation. Electronic claims are then produced with a few keystrokes, eliminating the need to repeatedly key patient information. This information is now stored in the EHR program.
- **Report generators**—these generators produce reports automatically by inserting required parameters rather than compiling data by hand.
- **Electronic prescriptions**—prescriptions can be produced by many EHR programs. These can be forwarded to the patient's pharmacy either electronically or by fax.
- **Ancillary service orders and results**—procedures such as X-rays and labs can be requested and results received via many EHR programs. Results coming from outside providers also can be scanned directly into the office EHR program as part of a patient's permanent record.
- **Patient portals**—more and more EHR programs are allowing patients access to certain portions of their medical records through an office patient portal. The portal allows patients to view routine information and perform routine tasks, such as making appointments, accessing a child's immunization record, or even paying balances on an account online.

General Rules When Working with EHR Programs

- Familiarize yourself with the program so that you can remain focused on the patient when entering data into the electronic health record.
- When retrieving an EHR, make sure you have identified the patient with at least two identifiers, such as name, date of birth, and/or medical record number.
- Keep your password information secure. Change the password often according to office policy.
- Keep the computer that contains the EHR secure, and back it up often.
- Carefully check your entry before submitting; EHR are legal documents.

Legal and Ethical Issues, Including HIPAA

4 Cs of Medical Malpractice Prevention

1. **Caring**—showing patients that you care about them may result in an improvement in their medical condition and, if you are sincere, decreases the likelihood that patients will feel the need to sue if treatment has unsatisfactory results or adverse events occur.
2. **Communication**—if you communicate in a professional manner and clearly ask for confirmation that you have been understood, you will earn respect and trust from your patients and other members of the allied health team.
3. **Competence**—be competent in your skills and job knowledge, and maintain and update your knowledge and skills frequently through continuing education.

4. **Charting**—documentation is proof of competence. Make sure that all current reports and consultations have been reviewed by the physician and are evident in the chart. Chart every conversation or interaction you have with a patient.

Credit and Collection Laws

Law	Requirements
Equal Credit Opportunity Act (ECOA)	• Creditors may not discriminate against applicants on the basis of sex, marital status, race, national origin, religion, or age. • Creditors may not discriminate because an applicant receives public assistance income or has exercised rights under the Consumer Credit Protection Act.
Fair Credit Reporting Act (FCRA)	This act requires credit bureaus to supply correct and complete information to businesses to use in evaluating a person's application for credit, insurance, or a job.
Fair Debt Collection Practices Act (FDCPA)	This act requires debt collectors to treat debtors fairly. It prohibits certain collection tactics, such as harassment, false statements, threats, and unfair practices.
Genetic Information Nondiscrimination Act (GINA)	This act protects individuals from discrimination based on their genetic information.
Truth in Lending Act (TILA)	This act requires creditors to provide applicants with accurate and complete credit costs and terms.

HIPAA and Patient Rights

- Patients have the right to choose a licensed practitioner.
- Patients also have the right to terminate a practitioner's services.

HIPAA Definitions

Use

Performing any of the following actions to individually identifiable health information by employees or other members of an organization's workforce:

- Sharing
- Employing
- Applying
- Utilizing
- Examining
- Analyzing

Disclosure

Performing any of the following actions so that the information is outside the entity:

- Releasing
- Transferring
- Providing access to
- Divulging in any manner

Information is disclosed when it is transmitted between or among organizations.

HIPAA "Do's and Don'ts"—When and What to Disclose

1. When in doubt about whether to release information, it is better not to release it.

2. It is the patient's, not the physician's, right to keep patient information confidential. If the patient wants to disclose the information, it is unethical for the physician not to do so.

3. All patients should be treated with the same degree of confidentiality, regardless of the healthcare professional's personal opinion of the patient.

4. You should be aware of all applicable laws and regulations of agencies such as public health departments.

5. When it is necessary to break confidentiality or when there is a conflict between ethics and confidentiality, discuss it with the patient. If the law does not dictate what to do in the situation, the attending physician should make the judgment based on the urgency of the situation and any danger that might be posed to the patient or others.

6. Get written approval from the patient before releasing information. For common situations, the patient should sign a standard release-of-records form.

HIPAA Security Rule

- A security officer must be assigned the responsibility for the medical facility's security.
- All staff, including management, receives security awareness training.

- Medical facilities must implement audit controls to record and examine staff who have logged in to information systems that contain PHI.
- Organizations limit physical access to medical facilities that contain electronic PHI.
- Organizations must conduct risk analyses to determine information security risks and vulnerabilities.
- Organizations must establish policies and procedures that allow access to electronic PHI on a need-to-know basis.

HIPAA Privacy Rule

- The core of the Privacy Rule is the protection, use, and disclosure of protected health information (PHI). This rule protects individuals' medical records and other personal health information, also known as individually identifiable health information (IIHI).

HITECH

- Stands for Health Information Technology for Economic and Clinical Health
- Increased privacy regulations by DHHS, particularly surrounding EHR
- Strengthens enforcement penalties relating to PHI breaches with EHR and practice management systems

PHI (IIHI)

- Name
- Address
- Phone numbers
- Fax number
- Dates (birth, death, admission, discharge, etc.)
- Social Security number
- E-mail address

- Medical record numbers
- Health plan beneficiary numbers
- Account numbers
- Certificate or license numbers
- Vehicle identifiers and serial numbers, including license plate numbers
- Device identifiers and serial numbers
- Web Uniform Resource Locators (URLs)
- Internet Protocol (IP) address numbers

Chart security

- Charts that contain a patient's name or other identifiers cannot be in view at the front reception area or in clinical areas. Some offices have placed charts in plain jackets to prevent information from being seen.
- Charts must be stored out of the view of a public area so that they cannot be seen by unauthorized individuals.
- Charts should be placed on the filing shelves without the patient name showing.
- Charts should be locked when not in use. Many facilities have purchased filing equipment that can be locked and unlocked without limiting the availability of patient information.
- Every staff member who uses patient information must be logged and a confidentiality statement signed. Signatures of staff should be on file with the office.

Patient care area security

- Log off or turn your monitor off when leaving your terminal or computer.
- When placing charts in exam room racks or in shelves, the name of the patient or other identifiers must be concealed from other patients.

- HIPAA does not have a regulation about calling patients' names in the reception area, but to increase privacy in your facility, you may suggest a numbering system to identify patients.
- When discussing a patient with another staff member or with the practitioner, make sure your voice is lowered and that all doors to the exam rooms are closed. Avoid discussing patient conditions in heavy traffic areas.
- When discussing a condition with a patient, make sure that you are in a private room or area where no one can hear you.
- Avoid discussing patients in lunchrooms, hallways, or any other place in a medical facility where someone can overhear you.

Copier security

- Do not leave confidential documents anywhere on the copier where others can read the information.
- Do not discard copies in a shared trash container; shred them.
- If a paper jam occurs, be sure to remove from the copier the copy or partial copy that caused the jam. If the copy contains PHI, shred it.

Fax security

- **Fax cover page**—state clearly on the fax cover sheet that confidential and protected health information is included. Further state that the information included is to be protected and must not be shared or disclosed without the appropriate authorizations from the patient.
- **Location of the fax machine**—keep the fax machine in an area that is not accessible by individuals who are not authorized to view PHI.

- **Faxes with protected health information**—faxes with PHI that your office receives must be stored promptly in a protected, secure area.
- **Fax number**—always confirm the accuracy of fax numbers to minimize the possibility of faxes being sent to the wrong person. Call people to tell them the fax is being sent.
- **Confirmation**—program the fax machine to print a confirmation for all faxes sent, and staple the confirmation sheet to each document sent.
- **Training**—train all staff members to understand the importance of safeguarding PHI sent or received via fax.

Printer security

- Do not print confidential material on a printer shared by other departments or in an area when others can read the material.
- Do not leave a printer unattended while printing confidential material.
- Before leaving the printing area, check to be sure all computer disks containing confidential information and all printed material have been collected.
- Be certain that the print job is sent to the right printer location.
- Do not discard printouts in a shared trash container; shred them.

Reception area security

- Log off or turn your monitor off when leaving your terminal or computer.
- The computer must be placed in an area where other patients cannot see the screen.

- Patient sign-in sheets may be used but must not include the reason for or nature of the patient visit. Likewise, patient names may be called out as long as no reference to the reason for the visit is made.

- Call centers and reception area phone conversations must be kept confidential. Many offices use sliding glass windows to allow for privacy when on the phone with other patients or offices.

Appendix I
Abbreviations

a before

$\overline{aa}$, $\overline{AA}$ of each

ABGs arterial blood gases

a.c. before meals

ADD attention deficit disorder

ADL activities of daily living

ad lib as desired

ADT admission, discharge, transfer

AIDS acquired immunodeficiency syndrome

AKA above knee amputation

a.m.a. against medical advice

AMA American Medical Association

amp. ampule

amt amount

aq., AQ water; aqueous

ausc. auscultation

ax axis

Bib, bib drink

b.i.d., bid, BID twice a day

BKA below knee amputation

BM bowel movement

BP, B/P blood pressure

BPC blood pressure check

BPH benign prostatic hypertrophy

BSA body surface area

$\overline{c}$ with

Ca, CA calcium; cancer

CABG coronary artery bypass graft

cap, caps capsules

CBC complete blood (cell) count

C.C., CC chief complaint

CDC Centers for Disease Control and Prevention

CHF congestive heart failure

chr chronic

cm centimeter

CNS central nervous system

Comp, comp compound

COPD chronic obstructive pulmonary disease

CP chest pain

CPE complete physical exam

CPR cardiopulmonary resuscitation

CSF cerebrospinal fluid

CT computed tomography

CV cardiovascular

CVA cerebrovascular accident

CXR chest X-ray

d day

D&C dilation and curettage

DEA Drug Enforcement Administration

Dil, dil dilute

DM diabetes mellitus

DNR do not resuscitate

DOB date of birth

Dr. doctor

DTaP diphtheria-tetanus-acellular pertussis

DTs delirium tremens

DVT deep venous thrombosis

D/W dextrose in water

Dx, dx diagnosis

ECG, EKG electrocardiogram

ED emergency department

EEG electroencephalogram

EENT eyes, ears, nose, and throat

EHR electronic health record

EMR electronic medical record

EP established patient

ER emergency room

ESR erythrocyte sedimentation rate

FBS fasting blood sugar

FDA Food and Drug Administration

FH family history

Fl, fl, fld fluid

fl oz fluid ounce

F/u, F/U, f/u follow-up

FUO fever of unknown origin

Fx fracture

g gram

GBS gallbladder series

GI gastrointestinal

Gm, gm gram

gr grain

gt, gtt drop(s)

GTT glucose tolerance test

GU genitourinary

GYN gynecology

HA headache

HB, Hgb hemoglobin

hct hematocrit

HEENT head, eyes, ears, nose, throat

HIV human immunodeficiency virus

HO history of

HPI history of present illness

HPV human papillomavirus

Hx history

ICU intensive care unit

I&D incision and drainage

I&O intake and output

IDDM insulin-dependent diabetes mellitus

IIHI individually identifiable health information

IM intramuscular

inf. infusion; inferior

inj injection

IT inhalation therapy

IUD intrauterine device

IV intravenous

KUB kidneys, ureters, bladder

L liter

L1, L2, etc. lumbar vertebrae

lab laboratory

lb pound

liq liquid

LLE left lower extremity (left leg)

LLL left lower lobe

LLQ left lower quadrant

LMP last menstrual period

LUE left upper extremity (left arm)

LUQ left upper quadrant

m meter

M mix (Latin *misce*)

mcg microgram

mg milligram

MI myocardial infarction

mL milliliter

mm millimeter

MM mucous membrane

mm Hg millimeters of mercury

MRI magnetic resonance imaging

MS multiple sclerosis

NB newborn

NED no evidence of disease

NIDDM noninsulin-dependent diabetes mellitus

no., # number

noc, noct night

npo, NPO nothing by mouth

NPT new patient

NS normal saline

NSAID nonsteroidal anti-inflammatory drug

NTP normal temperature and pressure

N&V nausea and vomiting

NYD not yet diagnosed

OB obstetrics

OC oral contraceptive

oint ointment

OOB out of bed

OPD outpatient department

OPS outpatient services

OR operating room

OT occupational therapy

OTC over-the-counter (medication)

oz ounce

p̄ after

P&P Pap smear (Papanicolaou smear) and pelvic exam

PA posteroanterior

Pap Pap smear

Path pathology

p.c., pc after meals

PE physical exam

per by, with

PFSH past family and/or social history

PH past history

PHI protected health information

PID pelvic inflammatory disease

PMS premenstrual syndrome

po by mouth

p/o postoperative

POMR problem-oriented medical record

p.r.n., prn, PRN whenever necessary

pt pint

Pt patient

PT physical therapy

PTA prior to admission

pulv powder

PVC premature ventricular contraction

q. every

q2, q2h every 2 hours

q.a.m., qam every morning

q.h., qh every hour

qns, QNS quantity not sufficient

qs, QS quantity sufficient

qt quart

RA rheumatoid arthritis; right atrium

RBC red blood cells; red blood (cell) count

RDA recommended dietary allowance, recommended daily allowance

REM rapid eye movement

RF rheumatoid factor

RLE right lower extremity (right leg)

RLL right lower lobe

RLQ right lower quadrant

R/O rule out

ROM range of motion

ROS/SR review of systems/systems review

RUE right upper extremity (right arm)

RUQ right upper quadrant

RV right ventricle

Rx prescription, take

$\overline{s}$ without

SAD seasonal affective disorder

SIDS sudden infant death syndrome

sig sigmoidoscopy

Sig directions

SL sublingual

SOAP subjective, objective, assessment, plan

SOB shortness of breath

sol solution

SOMR source-oriented medical record

S/R suture removal

Staph staphylococcus

stat, STAT immediately

STI sexually transmitted infection

Strep streptococcus

subcut, subcu, subQ subcutaneous

subling sublingual

surg surgery

S/W saline in water

SX symptoms

T1, T2, etc. thoracic vertebrae

T&A tonsillectomy and adenoidectomy

tab tablet

TB tuberculosis

tbs., tbsp tablespoon

TIA transient ischemic attack

t.i.d., tid, TID three times a day

tinc, tinct, tr tincture

TMJ temporomandibular joint

top topically

TPR temperature, pulse, and respiration

TSH thyroid-stimulating hormone

tsp teaspoon

Tx treatment

U unit

UA urinalysis

UCHD usual childhood diseases

UGI upper gastrointestinal

ung, ungt ointment

URI upper respiratory infection

US ultrasound

UTI urinary tract infection

VA visual acuity

VD venereal disease

VF visual field

VS vital signs

WBC white blood cells; white blood (cell) count

WNL within normal limits

wt weight

y/o year old

Appendix II
Medical Notation Symbols

Weights and Measures

#	pounds
°	degrees
′	foot; minute
″	inch; second
mEq	milliequivalent
mL	milliliter
dL	deciliter
mg%	milligrams percent; milligrams per 100 mL

Mathematical Functions and Terms

#	number
+	plus; positive; acid reaction
−	minus; negative; alkaline reaction
±	plus or minus; either positive or negative; indefinite
×	multiply; magnification; crossed with, hybrid
÷, /	divided by
=	equal to
≈	approximately equal to
>	greater than; from which is derived
<	less than; derived from
≮	not less than
≯	not greater than
≤	equal to or less than
≥	equal to or greater than

$\neq$	not equal to
$\sqrt{}$	square root
$\sqrt[3]{}$	cube root
∞	infinity
:	ratio; "is to"
$\therefore$	therefore
%	percent
π	pi (3.14159)—the ratio of the circumference of a circle to its diameter

Chemical Notations

Δ	change; heat
$\rightleftharpoons$	reversible reaction
$\uparrow$	increase
$\downarrow$	decrease

Warnings

$\mathbb{C}$	Schedule I controlled substance
$\mathbb{C}$	Schedule II controlled substance
$\mathbb{C}$	Schedule III controlled substance
$\mathbb{C}$	Schedule IV controlled substance
$\mathbb{C}$	Schedule V controlled substance
☠	poison
☢	radiation
☣	biohazard

Others

Rx	prescription; take
□, ♂	male
○, ♀	female
†	one
††	two
†††	three

Appendix III
Commonly Misspelled Terms

A. Medical Terms

abdominal	Alzheimer's
anergic	anesthetic
aneurysm	anteflexion
arrhythmia	asepsis
asthma	auricle
benign	bilirubin
bronchial	calcaneus
capillary	cervical
chancre	choroid
chromosome	cirrhosis
clavicle	curettage
cyanosis	defibrillator
desiccation	diluent
dissect	eosinophil
epididymis	epistaxis
erythema	eustachian
fissure	flexure
fomites	glaucoma
glomerular	gonorrhea
hemocytometer	hemorrhage

hemorrhoids	homeostasis
humerus	ileum
ilium	infarction
inoculate	intussusception
ischemia	ischium
larynx	leukemia
leukocyte	malaise
menstruation	metastasis
muscle	neuron
nosocomial	occlusion
ophthalmology	oscilloscope
osseous	palliative
parasite	parenteral
parietal	paroxysm
pericardium	perineum
peristalsis	peritoneum
pharynx	pituitary
plantar	pleurisy
pneumonia	polyp
prescription	prophylaxis
prostate	prosthesis
pruritus	psoriasis
psychiatrist	pyrexia
respiration	rheumatoid arthritis
schizophrenia	sciatic nerve
roentgenology	scirrhous
serous	specimen
sphincter	sphygmomanometer

squamous	staphylococcus
surgeon	vaccine
vein	venous
ventilator	wheal

B. Other Terms

absence	accept
accessible	accommodate
accumulate	achieve
acquire	adequate
advantageous	affect
aggravate	all right
a lot	already
altogether	analysis
analyze	apparatus
apparent	appearance
appropriate	approximate
argument	assistance
associate	auxiliary
balloon	bankruptcy
believe	benefited
brochure	bulletin
business	category
changeable	characteristic
cigarette	circumstance
clientele	committee
comparative	complement

compliment	concede
conscientious	conscious
controversy	corroborate
counsel	courtesy
defendant	definite
dependent	description
desirable	development
dilemma	disappear
disappoint	disapprove
disastrous	discreet
discrete	discrimination
dissatisfied	dissipate
earnest	ecstasy
effect	eligible
embarrass	emphasis
entrepreneur	envelope
environment	exceed
except	exercise
exhibit	exhilaration
existence	fantasy
fascinate	February
fluorescent	forty
grammar	grievance
guarantee	handkerchief
height	humorous
hygiene	incidentally
indispensable	inimitable

insistent	irrelevant
irresistible	irritable
its	it's
labeled	laboratory
led	leisure
liable	liaison
license	liquefy
maintenance	maneuver
miscellaneous	misspelled
necessary	noticeable
occasion	occurrence
offense	oscillate
paid	pamphlet
panicky	paradigm
parallel	paralyze
pastime	persevere
persistent	personal
personnel	persuade
phenomenon	plagiarism
pleasant	possession
precede	precedent
predictable	predominant
prejudice	preparation
prerogative	prevalent
principal	principle
privilege	procedure
proceed	professor

pronunciation	psychiatry
psychology	pursue
questionnaire	rearrange
recede	receive
recommend	referral
relieve	repetition
rescind	resume
rhythm	ridiculous
schedule	secretary
seize	separate
similar	sizable
stationary	stationery
stomach	subpoena
succeed	suddenness
supersede	surprise
tariff	technique
temperament	temperature
thorough	transferred
truly	tyrannize
unnecessary	until
vacillate	vacuum
vegetable	vicious
warrant	Wednesday
weird	

Appendix IV
Medical Terminology

NOTE: When referencing this appendix, note that some word parts are used in more than one way. For example, "cyt" serves as a word root in "cytology" but as a suffix in "astrocyte." If you do not initially find the word part you are looking for, check the other sections of this appendix to see if it is listed as another type of word part.

A. Prefixes

Prefix	Meaning
a-, an-	without, not
ab-	from, away
acr-, acro-	extremity, topmost
ad-	to, toward
ambi-, amph-, amphi-	both, on both sides, around
ante-	before
antero-	in front of
anti-	against, opposing
aque-	water
astro-	star-like
auto-	self
bi-	twice, double
brachy-	short

continued

Prefix	Meaning
brady-	slow
carboxy-	containing carbon and oxygen or a carboxyl group
cata-	down, lower, under
centi-	hundred
cephal-	head
chol-, chole-, cholo-	gall
chromo-	color
circum-	around
co-, com-, con-	together, with
contra-	against
cryo-	cold
crypt-, crypto-	hidden
cyan-, cyano-	blue
de-	down, from
deca-	ten
deci-	tenth
demi-	half
dextro-	to the right
di-	double, twice
dia-	through, apart, between
dipla-, diplo-	double, twin
dis-	apart, away from
dys-	difficult, painful, bad, abnormal
e-, ec-, ecto-	away, from, without, outside

Prefix	Meaning
echo-	sound, sound wave
electro-	electric
em-, en-	in, into, inside
endo-	within, inside
ento-	within, inner
epi-	on, above
erythro-	red
eu-	good
ex-, exo-	outside of, beyond, without
excori-	scratch or abrasion, loss of skin
extra-	outside of, beyond, in addition
fore-	before, in front of
glauc-, glauco-	gray
gyn-, gyno-, gyne-, gyneco-	woman, female
hemi-	half
hetero-	other, unlike
homeo-, homo-	same, like
hyper-	above, over, increased, excessive
hypo-	below, under, decreased
idio-	personal, self-produced
im-, in-, ir-	not
in-	in, into
inferi-	below

continued

Prefix	Meaning
infra-	beneath
inter-	between, among
intra-, intro-	into, within, during
juxta-	near, nearby
kata-, kath-	down, lower, under
kineto-	motion
leuco-, leuko-	white
levo-	to the left
macro-	large, long
mal-	bad
mega-, megalo-	large, great
meio-	contraction
melan-, melano-	black
membran-	pertaining to a membrane
mes-, meso-	middle
metr-, metro-	pertaining to the uterus
meta-	beyond
micro-	small
mid-	middle
mio-	smaller, less
mono-	single, one
multi-	many
neo-	new
non-, not-	no

Prefix	Meaning
nulli-	none
ob-	against
olig-, oligo-	few, less than normal
ortho-	straight
oxy-	sharp, acid
pachy-	thick
pan-	all, every
par-, para-	alongside of, with; woman who has given birth
per-	through, excessive
peri-	around
pes-	foot
pluri-	more, several
pneo-	breathing
poly-	many, much
post-, posteri-	after, behind
pre-, pro-	before, in front of
presby-, presbyo-	old age
primi-	first
pseudo-	false
quadri-	four
re-	back, again
retro-	backward, behind
semi-	half

continued

Prefix	Meaning
steno-	contracted, narrow
stereo-	firm, solid, three-dimensional
sub-	under
super-, supra-	above, upon, excess
sym-, syn-	with, together
tachy-	fast
tele-	distant, far
tetra-	four
tomo-	incision, section
trans-	across
tri-	three
tropho-	nutrition, growth
ultra-	beyond, excess
uni-	one
veni-	vein
xanth-, xantho-	yellow

B. Suffixes

Suffix	Meaning
-ad	to, toward
-aesthesia, -esthesia	sensation
-al	characterized by, pertaining to
-algia	pain

Suffix	Meaning
-ase	enzyme
-asthenia	weakness
-cele	swelling, tumor
-centesis	puncture, tapping
-ceps	heads
-cidal	killing
-cide	causing death
-cise	cut
-clast	to break
-coele	cavity
-crine	to excrete
-cyst	bladder, bag
-cyte	cell, cellular
-duction	to pull or move
-dynia	pain
-ectomy	cutting out, surgical removal
-edema	fluid buildup
-emesis	vomiting
-emia	blood
-esthesia	sensation
-extension	increasing the angle of a joint
-flexion	bending
-form	shape

continued

Suffix	Meaning
-fuge	driving away
-gen, -genesis, -gon	born, produced
-gene, -genic, -genetic, -genesis, -genous	arising from, origin, formation
-glia	pertaining to glial cells
-globin, -globulin	protein
-gram	recorded information
-graph	instrument for recording
-graphy	the process of recording
-ia	condition
-iasis	condition of
-ic, -ical	pertaining to
-ician	specialist in a field
-id	having the characteristics of
-ism	condition, process, theory
-itis	inflammation of
-ium	membrane
-ive	with the properties of
-ize	to cause to be, to become, to treat by special method
-kinesis, -kinetic	motion
-lepsis, -lepsy	seizure, convulsion
-lith	stone
-logy	science of, study of

Suffix	Meaning
-lysis	setting free, disintegration, decomposition
-malacia	abnormal softening
-mania	insanity, abnormal desire
-megaly	enlargement
-meter	measure
-metrist	one who measures
-metry	process of measuring
-motor	movement
-odynia	pain
-oid	resembling
-ole	small, little
-oma	tumor
-opia	vision
-opsy	to view
-osis	disease, condition of
-or	relating to
-ostomy	to make a mouth, opening
-otomy	incision, surgical cutting
-ous	having
-pathy	disease, suffering
-pelvic	pelvis
-penia	too few, lack, decreased
-pexy	surgical fixation

continued

Suffix	Meaning
-phagia, -phage	eating, consuming, swallowing
-phobia	fear, abnormal fear
-phylaxis	protection
-plasia	formation or development
-plastic	molded
-plasty	operation to reconstruct, surgical repair
-plegia	paralysis
-pnea	breathing
-poiesis	to make or produce
-ptysis	spitting
-rrhage, -rrhagia	abnormal or excessive discharge, hemorrhage, flow
-receptor	cell that can send a signal to the brain
-rrhaphy	suture of
-rrhea	flow, discharge
-sarcoma	malignant tumor
-sclerosis	hardening
-scope	instrument used to examine
-scopy	examining
-sepsis	poisoning, infection
-spasm	cramp or twitching
-stasis	stoppage
-stalsis	contraction

Suffix	Meaning
-stomy	opening
-thalamus	pertaining to the thalamus
-therapy	treatment
-thermy	heat
-thorax	chest
-tome	cutting instrument
-tomy	incision, section
-tory	pertaining to
-toxic	poison
-tripsy	surgical crushing
-trophy	turning, tendency
-tropic	in response to a stimulus
-tropy	turning, tendency
-ula, -ule	little
-uria	urine
-uretic	pertaining to urine
-verse, -version	turned or directed

C. Word Roots

Word Root	Meaning
abdomino-	abdomen
adeno-	gland, glandular

continued

Word Root	Meaning
adipo-	fat
adreno-	adrenal glands
aero-	air
andr-, andro-	man, male
ambly-	dull, dim
angio-	blood vessel
ano-	anus
anthrac-, anthraco-	coal, carbon
arterio-	artery
arthro-	joint
athero-	soft, fatty deposit
atrio-	pertaining to the atria of the heart
audi-	hearing
baro-	weight, pressure
bili-	bile
bio-	life
blasto-, blast-	developing stage, bud, immature
bracheo-	arm
broncho-	bronchial (windpipe)
burs-	bursa
carcino-	cancer
cardio-	heart

Word Root	Meaning
caud-	tail
cellul-	cells
cerebr-, cerebro-	brain
cephalo-	head
cervico-	neck
chondro-	cartilage
chromo-	color
colo-	colon
colp-, colpo-	vagina
conjunctiv-	conjunctiva
coro-	body
cortico-	cortex
cost-, costo-	rib
cox-	hip
crani-, cranio-	skull
cusp-	projection
cysto-	bladder, bag
cyto-	cell, cellular
dacry-, dacryo-	tears, lacrimal apparatus
dactyl-, dactylo-	finger, toe
dent-, denti-, dento-	teeth
derma-, dermat-, dermato-	skin
dist-	farthest from the point of attachment

continued

Word Root	Meaning
diverticul-	diverticula
dorsi-, dorso-	back
dur-, dura-	pertaining to the dura mater of the brain
encephalo-	brain
entero-	intestine
episi-, episio-	pertaining to the pubic region
esophag-	esophagus
esthesio-	sensation
femor-	femur
fibro-	connective tissue
follicul-	follicle
front-	forehead
galact-, galacto-	milk
gastr-, gastro-	stomach
gingiv-	gums
glomerulo-	glomerulus
glosso-	tongue
gluco-, glyco-	sugar, sweet
granulo-	granules
gravid-, gravid-	pregnant female
haemo-, hemato-, hem-, hemo-	blood
hepa-, hepar-, hepato-	liver
herni-	rupture

Word Root	Meaning
hidro-	sweat (perspiration)
histo-	tissue
hydra-, hydro-	water
hyster-, hystero-	uterus
ictero-	jaundice
ileo-	ileum
immuno-	pertaining to the immune system
interstit-	interstices
karyo-	nucleus, nut
kera-, kerato-	horn, hardness, cornea
keratino-	keratin
labyrinth-	pertaining to the labyrinth of the ears
lacrim-, lacrimo-	tears
lact-, lactifer-	milk
laparo-	abdomen
laryngo-	pertaining to the larynx
later-, latero-	side
linguo-	tongue
lipo-	fat
lith-	stone
lobo-	lobe
lun-, luna-	moon

continued

Word Root	Meaning
lymph-, lympho-	lymphatic, spring water
mast-, masto-	breast
med-, medi-	middle
mening-	meninges (covers the brain)
metacarpo-	pertaining to the metacarpal bones
metatarso-	pertaining to the metatarsal bones
metro-, metra-	uterus
my-, myo-	muscle
myel-, myelo-	marrow
narco-	sleep
nas-, naso-	nose
nat-, nato-	born
natri-	sodium
necro-	dead
nephr-, nephro-	kidney
neu-, neuro-	nerve
niter-, nitro-	nitrogen
nucleo-	nucleus
oculo-	eye
odont-	tooth
omphalo-	navel, umbilicus
onco-	tumor

Word Root	Meaning
onych-, onycho-	pertaining to the nail of a finger or toe
oo-	ovum, egg
ov-, ovi-, ovo-	pertaining to an ovum or egg
oophor-	ovary
ophthalmo-	eye
opt-, opto-	vision
orchid-	testicle
or-, oro-	pertaining to the mouth
os-	mouth, opening
oste-, osteo-	bone
oto-	ear
paedo-, pedo-	child
palpebro-	eyelid
pancrea-	pancreas
path-, patho-	disease, suffering
pedicul-	lice
pepso-	digestion
peptid-	pertaining to a peptide
phag-, phago-	eating, consuming, swallowing
phalang-	pertaining to the phalanges
pharyng-, pharyngo-	throat, pharynx
phlebo-	vein

continued

Word Root	Meaning
photo-	pertaining to light
pleuro-	side, rib
pneumo-	air, lungs
pod-	foot
procto-	rectum
proxim-	close to the point of attachment
psych-	the mind
pulmon-, pulmono-	lung
pyelo-	pelvis (renal)
pylor-	pylorus (part of the stomach)
pyo-, pus-	pus
pyro-	fever, heat
refract-	refraction, refractive
reni-, reno-	kidney
retino-	retina
rhabdo-	rod-shaped
rhino-	nose
sacchar-	sugar
sacro-	sacrum
sagitt-	dividing into left and right
salpingo-	tube, fallopian tube
sarco-	flesh
sclero-	hard, sclera

Word Root	Meaning
scolio-	lateral curvature
sebace-	oil
sensori-	the senses
sigmo-	S-shaped
septi-, septic-, septico-	poison, infection
som-, soma-	body
sperma-, spermato-	semen, spermatozoa
spleno-	spleen
steroid-	steroid (lipid-soluble substance)
stomato-	mouth
synapt-	pertaining to a synapse
synov-	synovium
sudorifer-	sweat
superfic-	near the surface
superi-	above
tempor-	pertaining to the temple
teno-, tenoto-, tendon-	tendon
thermo-	heat
thio-	sulfa
thoraco-	chest
thrombo-	blood clot
thymo-	thymus
thyro-	thyroid gland

continued

Word Root	Meaning
tricho-	hair
tubulo-	tube, tubule
tympan-	eardrum
ureth-	urethra
urino-, uro-	urine, urinary organs
utero-	uterus, uterine
uvulo-	uvula
vagin-	vagina
vaso-, vasculo-	vessel
ventr-	front
ventricul-, ventriculo-	pertaining to the ventricles of the heart
ventri-, ventro-	abdomen
vesico-	blister
vulvo-	pertaining to the vulva

Appendix V
Common Spanish Phrases

English Phrase	Spanish Translation and Pronunciation
Do you speak English?	¿Habla usted inglés? *AH-blah ooh-STEHD een-GLAYSS*
Do you understand English?	¿Entiende usted inglés? *en-tee-EN-day ooh-STEHD een-GLAYSS*
I do not speak Spanish well.	Yo no hablo español bien. *yo no AH-bloh ess-pan-YOHL bee-YEN*
Please speak more slowly.	Hable más despacio, por favor. *AH-blay mahss deh-SPAH-see-yoh pore fah-VOHR*
Please repeat.	Repita, por favor. *ray-PEE-tah pore fah-VOHR*
I don't understand.	No entiendo. No comprendo. *no en-tee-EN-doh. No kom-PREN-doh*

continued

English Phrase	Spanish Translation and Pronunciation
Are you a family member?	¿Es usted miembro de la familia? *ess ooh-STEHD mee-EM-broh day lah fah-MEE-lee-yah*
Are you a friend of the family?	¿Es usted amigo (*if the person is male*)/amiga (*if the person is female*) de la familia? *ess ooh-STEHD ah-MEE-goh/ ah-MEE-gah day lah fah-MEE-lee-yah*
Can you interpret for me (us)?	¿Puede servir de intérprete? *PWAY-day sehr-VEER day in-TAYR-pray-tay*
Can you translate?	¿Puede traducir? *PWAY-day trah-due-SEER*
Have you been ill?	¿Usted ha estado enfermo (*when speaking to a male*)/ enferma (*when speaking to a female*)? *ooh-STEHD ah ess-TAH-doh en-FAYR-moh/en-FAYR-mah*
What is your full name?	¿Cuál es su nombre completo? *kwall ess soo NOME-bray kom-PLAY-toh*
What is your date of birth?	¿Cuál es la fecha de su nacimiento? *kwall ess lah FAY-cha day soo nah-see-mee-EN-toh*

English Phrase	Spanish Translation and Pronunciation
What is your address?	¿Cuál es su dirección? *kwall es soo dee-rek-see-OWN*
What is your phone number?	¿Cuál es su número de teléfono? *kwall ess soo NEW-mehr-oh day tay-LAY-foh-noh*
What kind of pain do you have?	¿Cómo es su dolor? *KOH-mo ess soo doh-LOHR*
How do you feel today?	¿Cómo se siente hoy? *KOH-mo say see-EN-tay oy*
I am checking your pulse.	Estoy tomándole el pulso. *ess-TOY toh-MAHN-doh-lay ell POOL-soh*
I am checking your blood pressure.	Estoy tomándole la presión arterial. *ess-TOY toh-MAHN-doh-lay lah pray-see-OHN ahr-tayr-ee-AHL*
I need to listen to your heart and lungs.	Necesito escuchar su corazón y sus pulmones. *neh-seh-SEE-toh ess-koo-CHAR soo kor-ah-ZOHN ee soos pool-MOHN-ayss*
I need to touch you now.	Necesito palparlo ahora. *neh-seh-SEE-toh pal-PAR-loh ah-OH-rah*
Please open your shirt.	Por favor, ábrase la camisa. *pohr fah-VOHR AH-brah-say lah kah-MEE-sah*

continued

English Term	Spanish Translation and Pronunciation
yes	sí *see*
no	no *no*
maybe	quizás/tal vez *key-ZAHSS/tahl VAYSS*
up	arriba *ah-REE-bah*
down	abajo *ah-BAH-ho*
left	a la izquierda *a lah eez-kee-AIR-dah*
right	a la derecha *a lah deh-RAY-chah*
in	adentro *ah-DEN-troh*
out	afuera *ah-FWEH-rah*
around	alrededor *al-ray-day-DOOR*
above	sobre *SO-bray*
here	aquí *ah-KEE*

English Term	Spanish Translation and Pronunciation
there	allá *ah-YAH*
front	enfrente *en-FREN-tay*
back	detrás *day-TRAHS*
top	arriba *ah-REE-bah*
bottom	abajo *ah-BAH-ho*
I don't know	No sé. *No say*
Numbers:	**Números** ***NEW-mehr-ohss***
0	cero *SEH-roh*
1	uno *OO-noh*
2	*dos* *dohss*
3	*tres* *trayss*
4	cuatro *KWAH-troh*

continued

English Term	Spanish Translation and Pronunciation
5	cinco *SEEN-koh*
6	seis *sayss*
7	siete *see-YAY-tay*
8	ocho *OWE-choh*
9	nueve *new-AY-vay*
10	diez *dee-YAYSS*
11	once *OHN-say*
12	doce *DOH-say*
13	trece *TRAY-say*
14	catorce *kah-TOHR-say*
15	quince *KEEN-say*
16	dieciséis *dee-yayss-ee-SAYSS*

English Term	Spanish Translation and Pronunciation
17	diecisiete *dee-yayss-ee-see-YAY-tay*
18	dieciocho *dee-yayss-ee-OH-choh*
19	diecinueve *dee-yayss-ee-new-AY-vay*
20	veinte *BAYN-tay*
30	treinta *TRAYN-tah*
40	cuarenta *kwa-RAYN-tah*
50	cincuenta *sink-WAYN-tah*
60	sesenta *say-SAYN-tah*
70	setenta *say-TAYN-tah*
80	ochenta *owe-CHAYN-tah*
90	noventa *noh-BAYN-tah*
100	cien *see-EN*

continued

English Term	Spanish Translation and Pronunciation
Days of the week:	**Días de la semana** *DEE-ahs day lah say-MAH-nah*
Sunday	domingo *doh-MEEN-goh*
Monday	lunes *LOO-nayss*
Tuesday	martes *MAR-tayss*
Wednesday	miércoles *mee-YEHR-ko-layss*
Thursday	jueves *HWAY-vayss*
Friday	viernes *vee-YEHR-nayss*
Saturday	sábado *SAH-bah-doh*
Time References	**referencias tiempo** *Re-fe-REN-si-ahs ti-EM-po*
yesterday	ayer *ah-YEHR*
today	hoy *oy*
tomorrow	mañana *mah-NYAH-nah*

English Term	Spanish Translation and Pronunciation
this morning	esta mañana *ESS-tah mah-NYAH-na*
this afternoon	esta tarde *ESS-tah TAHR-day*
this evening	esta noche *ESS-tah NOH-chay*
day	día *DEE-ah*
week	semana *say-MAH-nah*
month	mes *mayss*
Months of the year:	**Meses del año:** ***MAY-sayss del AHN-yoh***
January	enero *eh-NAYR-oh*
February	febrero *feh-BRAYR-oh*
March	marzo *MAR-soh*
April	abril *ah-BREEL*
May	mayo *MY-oh*

continued

English Term	Spanish Translation and Pronunciation
June	junio *HOO-nee-oh*
July	julio *HOO-lee-oh*
August	agosto *ah-GOHS-toh*
September	septiembre *sep-tee-EM-bray*
October	octubre *ohk-TOO-bray*
November	noviembre *no-vee-EM-bray*
December	diciembre *dee-cee-EM-bray*
year	año *AH-nyoh*

Appendix VI
ASL American
Manual Alphabet

A
Palm is always
forward except
where noted

B

C
Palm forward
thumb bent out

D

E
Thumb also
often lower
(like a claw)

F

G
Palm in

H
Palm in

I

J

K

L

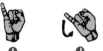

M

N

O
Palm faces
opposite side
of body

P
Index finger
points out

continued

311

Q
Like p but points down and unseen fingers curled in

R

S

T

U

V

W

X
Palm forward; thumb can be over fingers; whole palm can be slanted to side away from body

Y

Z

0

1

2

3

4

5

6

7

8

9

Appendix VII
Local Emergency and Contact Numbers

Alcohol and Drug Abuse Center _____

Behavioral Health _____

Children and Family Crisis Services _____

Community Health _____

Domestic Violence Hotline _____

Emergency Management and

Hazard Control _____

Government Offices _____

Hospice Care _____

Hospital(s) _____

Local Homeless Shelters _____

Local Red Cross _____

National Suicide Prevention Lifeline 800-273-TALK (8255)

Nonemergency Police _____

Poison Control Center 800-222-1222

    Local Number _____

Sexual Assault Hotline _____

Social Services _____

Translation Services _____

OTHER: _____

_____

_____

_____

Appendix VIII
Professional Medical Organizations

- American Academy of Professional Coders (AAPC:) http://www.aapc.com
- American Association of Medical Assistants (AAMA): http://www.aama-ntl.org
- American College of Physicians (ACP): http://www.acponline.org
- American Hospital Association (AHA): http://www.aha.org
- American Medical Association (AMA): http://www.ama-assn.org
- American Medical Billing Association (AMBA): http://www.ambanet.net
- American Medical Technologists (AMT): http://www.americanmedtech.org
- American Pharmacists Association (APhA): http://www.pharmacist.com
- American Society for Clinical Pathology (ASCP): http://www.ascp.org
- American Society of Phlebotomy Technicians (ASPT): http://www.aspt.org
- Association for Healthcare Documentation Integrity (AHDI): http://www.ahdionline.org
- National Association for Health Professionals (NAHP): http://www.nahpusa.com
- National Center for Competency Testing (NCCT): http://www.ncctinc.com

- National Healthcareer Association (NHA): http://www.nhanow.com
- National Occupational Competency Testing Institute (NOCTI): http://www.nocti.org

Appendix IX
Medical Resources on the Internet

- Academy of Nutrition and Dietetics—http://www.eatright.org
- American Cancer Society—http://www.cancer.org
- American Diabetes Association—http://www.diabetes.org
- American Heart Association—http://www.heart.org
- Anorexia Nervosa and Related Eating Disorders—http://www.anred.com
- Centers for Disease Control and Prevention—http://www.cdc.gov
- eMedicine Consumer Health—http://www.emedicinehealth.com/script/main/hp.asp
- Mayo Clinic—http://www.mayoclinic.org
- MedlinePlus—http://www.nlm.nih.gov/medlineplus
- National Association of Anorexia Nervosa and Associated Disorders—http://www.anad.org
- National Center for Complementary and Integrative Health—http://nccih.nih.gov
- National Eating Disorders Association—http://www.nationaleatingdisorders.org
- National Library of Medicine—http://www.nlm.nih.gov
- New England Journal of Medicine—http://www.nejm.org
- Occupational Safety and Health Administration—http://www.osha.gov
- Overeaters Anonymous (OA)—http://www.oa.org
- PDR Health—http://www.pdrhealth.com
- RXList—http://www.rxlist.com
- WebMD—http://www.webmd.com

Index